BROAI
REVEALED

BROADMOOR REVEALED

Victorian Crime and the Lunatic Asylum

Mark Stevens

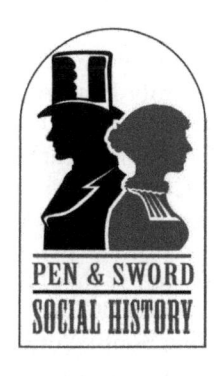

First published in Great Britain in 2013
and reprinted in this format in 2020 and 2021 by
PEN & SWORD SOCIAL HISTORY
an imprint of
Pen & Sword Books Ltd
47 Church Street
Barnsley
South Yorkshire
S70 2AS

Copyright © Mark Stevens, 2013, 2020, 2021

ISBN: 978 1 52679 647 9

The right of Mark Stevens to be identified as Author of this Work has been asserted by him in accordance with the Copyright, Designs and Patents Act 1988.

A CIP catalogue record for this book is available from the British Library.

All rights reserved. No part of this book may be reproduced or transmitted in any form or by any means, electronic or mechanical including photocopying, recording or by any information storage and retrieval system, without permission from the Publisher in writing.

Typeset in 11/13pt Palatino by
Concept, Huddersfield, West Yorkshire

Printed and bound in England by
CPI Group (UK) Ltd, Croydon, CR0 4YY

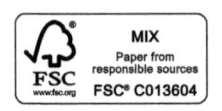

MIX
Paper from responsible sources
FSC® C013604

Pen & Sword Books Ltd incorporates the Imprints of Pen & Sword Aviation, Pen & Sword Family History, Pen & Sword Maritime, Pen & Sword Military, Pen & Sword Discovery, Wharncliffe Local History, Wharncliffe True Crime, Wharncliffe Transport, Pen & Sword Select, Pen & Sword Military Classics, Leo Cooper, The Praetorian Press, Remember When, Seaforth Publishing and Frontline Publishing.

For a complete list of Pen & Sword titles please contact
PEN & SWORD BOOKS LIMITED
47 Church Street, Barnsley, South Yorkshire, S70 2AS, England
E-mail: enquiries@pen-and-sword.co.uk
Website: www.pen-and-sword.co.uk

Contents

Acknowledgements		vi
Preface		viii
1	Broadmoor Hospital: By Way of Introduction	1
2	Edward Oxford: Shooting at Royalty	26
3	Richard Dadd: Artist of Repute	36
4	William Chester Minor: Man of Words and Letters	50
5	Broadmoor's International Brigade	64
6	Christiana Edmunds: The Venus of Broadmoor	93
7	Broadmoor Babies	108
8	Escape from Broadmoor	128
9	Only Passing Through	161
10	Sources	168
Index		174

Acknowledgements

There are lots of people to thank for helping to make this book a reality. First thanks should probably go to those people at Broadmoor who took an interest in the archive and thought that it was important. They include various people that I'd like to thank individually: Trevor Walt; Sheena Ebsworth; Kevin Murray; Robin Webster; as well as John Heritage and Bernard Foulness, who looked after the archive on site for many years. Then there are colleagues at the Berkshire Record Office who have helped to look after the archive once it came into our care: Peter Durrant; Sabina Sutherland; Sue Hourigan; Kate Tyte; and Rhonda Niven; as well as Glenn Bartley, who we commissioned to do some of the conservation work. That the archive is available in such a useful form is also due to the generosity of The Wellcome Trust. Special thanks go to Sue Crossley for that.

In terms of publication, I would like to thank first Andrzej Zychla of Mor-pho Publishing, who succeeded in creating the first hard copy edition of the book. It's in Polish and is probably all the better for it. Then thanks must go to Pen and Sword for taking a punt on a new edition of a work that had been given away free to over a quarter of a million people in the UK alone. Somehow they have managed to square commercial publishing with my public service values. I must also report that Jen Newby from Pen and Sword is a wonderfully straightforward and helpful person to work with and I commend her to anyone that she concerns.

I need to thank my family for not minding so many lunatics taking over their house. I fear that they may have to get used to it.

Acknowledgements

I should also thank all the fellow travellers that I have met along the way. There are many of you, but I must single out Leonora Klein, Geoffrey Munn, Richard Lansdown, Charlotte Edmunds and Steve Hennessy, who have all taken my own research further than it might otherwise have gone.

The final acknowledgement in this book needs to go to the people of Broadmoor, that is staff and patients, past and present, as well as their friends and families. And yes, anyone else who has been touched personally by a Broadmoor story in either a positive or a negative way. Broadmoor remembers you, always.

Preface

This book was intended to be a guide for researchers wanting to use the Broadmoor Hospital archive. The objective of the guide was to let people know that the archive existed, that it was stored at the Berkshire Record Office, and to suggest how its contents could be used to discover both the hospital and the patients who spent time within it. While the original objective survives, as my own research has developed so the book has become more of a travelogue than a trip advisor. The finished version seeks to hold your hand as it takes you round a gallery of the asylum's tourist sites, some well-known and others freshly discovered. It wants you to understand that you cannot take in all of Broadmoor with one glance. You must be led, and the individual views considered in context, if you wish to comprehend the whole.

This is not always a straightforward task. As you might expect, a lot of restrictions remain on access to the archive; in particular, patients' medical records are closed for a considerable time. This meant that the guide needed to focus on the Victorian period if it was to take some recognisable pictures, but even then obstructions might still partially obscure the view. Also, plenty of very interesting pathways from the period remain beyond reach for several years to come.

Because the guide was originally created as a series of online articles, it was not constructed in a linear fashion. I began by putting together biographies of those nineteenth century patients who are already part of public consciousness: Edward Oxford; Richard Dadd; William Chester Minor; and Christiana Edmunds.

Preface

They are four patients that others have already written about in more depth and with greater insight. However, they are also only four patients out of over 2,000 admitted before 1901, so for me, the more interesting thing became finding out the stories of those patients that I did not know. There is no shortage of such people. You could choose virtually any patient and find a fascinating personal history, which can also bring something new to our understanding of Victorian England and its care and management of the mentally ill.

I chose three areas to focus on. Firstly, I felt that the stories of the women of Broadmoor needed to be heard, and that Christiana Edmunds was too unusual a case to be representative of that group. On the other hand, a representative female case would have to be a child murderer – the most common reason for a female admission – and this would lack the redemptive element of the male stories of Oxford, Dadd and Minor, who were all remembered for achieving something despite their illnesses. I decided to balance my infanticide narrative by writing about the female patients who had experienced motherhood while in Broadmoor and the babies who came into the world through the asylum, as well as those who had left it.

Secondly, I wanted to report that not every patient in Broadmoor enjoyed the life advantages afforded to Dadd and Minor, both of whom came from educated, comfortable backgrounds. Many patients had lived a hand to mouth existence where dictionaries and drawing were absent luxuries. Finally, I considered that I should not shy away from the non-medical aim of the asylum as a place of public protection. Rather than dwell on tales of violence and destruction, I decided to discuss the concept through the medium of escape attempts. By writing about those that were successful or otherwise, I also hoped to dispel some of the preconceptions that exist about the dangers of an escaped lunatic.

This book has been put together from these individual pieces. There are many other topics that might be researched: the military and the British Empire, and the educated mad are two further chapters that one day I might get round to writing up. My interest in the hospital never seems to settle on one thing. In the meantime, I have two more books planned, both of which are intended to reveal more about Victorian Broadmoor. There is so much I could tell you about the place, but for now, perhaps I had best let you explore for yourself.

Mark Stevens
Reading, Berkshire
October 2012.

1

Broadmoor Hospital: By Way of Introduction

On 27 May 1863, three horse-drawn coaches pulled up at the gates of a recently-built national institution, set amongst the tall, dense pines of Windsor Forest. Inside the coaches were eight women and their escorts from Bethlem Hospital in London, the ancient hospital for the treatment of the insane. That morning the little party had left the Bethlem buildings in Southwark, boarded a train at Waterloo Station, then travelled by steam through the capital's suburbs and out to the little market town of Wokingham in Berkshire. Their destination was Broadmoor, England's first criminal lunatic asylum.

At half past twelve they had alighted from the train at Wokingham's simple railway station and found the large, grandly-titled Broadmoor Omnibus, together with two smaller, hired vehicles waiting to take them on the last leg of their journey. The eight women, their escorts and accompanying paperwork were loaded into the seats before the steps were removed, the doors fastened and the horses started. Then the wheels of the coaches spun down winding dirt track lanes and finally up a gentle incline, as the passengers were driven the five miles to the village of Crowthorne. Broadmoor's first patients had arrived.

Who were these women who had left their cramped confines in London for rural Berkshire? As befitted a group thrown together by circumstance, they had a mix of different backgrounds. One was a petty thief from Cheshire, while another had stabbed her husband when they were out poaching near York. The other six had all shared a single life event, however. They had killed or wounded their own children; either strangling them, drowning them or cutting their throats with a razor.

One mother had slashed her newborn with a blade rather than suckle it; another, the wife of a steamboat captain, had taken her three boys down to the Thames and thrown them in. A matron of this group was the first patient to be listed in the asylum's brand new admissions register. Mary Ann Parr was about 35 years of age, and a labourer from Nottingham. She had lived in poverty all her life, almost certainly suffered from congenital syphilis, and had what we would now call learning disabilities. Mary might have eked out an existence as just another member of the industrial poor, except that when she was 25 years old she had given birth to an illegitimate child and then suffocated it against her breast. She was convicted of murder and sentenced to death, before her sentence was commuted first to transportation for life and then, after a medical examination, to treatment instead in Bethlem.

When Mary Ann Parr arrived at Broadmoor she went through the same procedure as every Victorian patient who came after her. Relevant details were recorded from the forms that accompanied her, and then she underwent a medical examination and an interview with one of the doctors. All the while notes were taken, and then written up into a large case book and added to over the years. An extract from the notes made about Mary Ann Parr on admission reads: 'A woman of weak intellect, complains of pains in the forehead, short stature, cataract of the left and right eyes – can see a little with the left eye only. Teeth irregular and notched...Of very irritable temper.' Once documented, the patient was taken off to the admissions ward, and their crime unlikely to be further mentioned.

The women were given the best treatment available at the time. This was rather different to how we might understand mental health treatment today: there were no drug therapies available during Victorian times, nor psychiatric analysis. Instead, Her Majesty's lunatics were subject to a regime known as 'moral treatment'. This was a recognisable Victorian asylum concept. All patients were given a daily routine of exercise and occupation (which for Mary Ann Parr meant working in the laundry); regular

Broadmoor Hospital: By Way of Introduction

meals of fairly bland food; and plenty of fresh air. Sedatives or stimulants were available to the medical staff, but otherwise the moral routine employed was intended to bring about a cure. The other intervention granted staff was giving patients relief from their immediate domestic surroundings. In the case of the indigent Mary Ann Parr, her quality of life inside the walls was probably significantly better than she had enjoyed outside: she had a roof over her head, and she did not have to worry about food or money. This was the asylum as refuge: by removing a patient from their day-to-day life, the Victorians believed they would be able to neutralise whatever factor was causing their insanity, leading to beneficial results. It was a recognition that community living could create problems as well as solutions.

Mary Ann Parr was a reasonably typical recipient of this treatment regime in that she experienced it for the next 37 years, until she died in 1900, aged 71, from kidney disease. Many patients spent decades on site and became institutionalised in the process, although this outcome was by no means a given. The discharge rate on the male side was around one in five, and even greater on the female side, with slightly more than one in three patients being discharged, though the greater proportion of these were simply moved on to other institutions. Discharge rates from Broadmoor were so high in part due to the patient make up. While those detained at Her Majesty's pleasure knew the outcome of their case lay ultimately with the Home Secretary, a significant proportion of patients arrived instead from the prison system with a fixed sentence that they were required to serve. Once that sentence was complete, they were usually discharged to a local asylum for care.

* * *

The fact of Broadmoor's opening does not directly explain the fact of Broadmoor's creation. Every story has a beginning, and in Broadmoor's case this is usually traced back to a spring day in 1800. On the evening of 15 May that year, King George III chose to attend the Theatre Royal in Drury Lane, only to feel the coarse whistle of two shots pass near his head as he was taking his seat in the royal box.

The assailant turned out to be a member of the audience. James Hadfield was a young father from London who had fought for King and country in the French Revolutionary Wars and suffered dreadful injuries in battle. He had returned from war a raving madman, and his fellow soldiers chained him to a cart in his Surrey barracks until his brother came to take him home. Hadfield was now in thrall to a millenarian cult and convinced that he needed to secure his own death at the hands of the state. By suffering the same fate as Christ, Hadfield believed that his personal sacrifice would benefit all mankind by ushering in the Second Coming and the Day of Judgement. His public-spirited motivation was lost on the crowd at Drury Lane. After he had climbed onto the bench seats to fire his pistols, Hadfield was restrained in the orchestra pit while pandemonium raged around him.

It was soon quite clear that Hadfield had lost all reason. Legally, though, he presented something of a problem. While he might be found not guilty by reason of insanity, historically this verdict was reserved for those described as 'brutes' or 'infants', who were either unable to experience a solitary lucid moment or incapable of caring for themselves. The usual result was a discharge, sometimes to Bethlem, more often to family or the local community for care, but certainly with no further attention from the state. This approach was considered to be extremely risky in Hadfield's case, as it seemed entirely plausible that if let go, he might try something similar again.

Besides, Hadfield was neither brute nor infant. He was married, a father, and in regular employment in the silver trade. He had plenty of periods of lucidity. His case bore similarities to those of two previous assailants on the royal person, Margaret Nicholson and John Frith, neither of which had been resolved satisfactorily from a legal point of view. Both had been useful members of society before their illnesses, and both were the recipients of rather bungled hearings before they were shuffled off to Bethlem. Frith and Nicholson would have been fresh in the minds of the lawyers brought in to deal with the war hero Hadfield. Now they had been presented with another opportunity to find a satisfactory way of managing the dangerous lunatic. Fortunately, because Hadfield had been charged with treason, the ancient statutes granted him a right to counsel, a right which was not automatic for other defendants at the time. This meant that there could be a proper argument in court.

Broadmoor Hospital: By Way of Introduction

An able lawyer, Thomas Erskine, was deliberately picked as Hadfield's champion because of his slightly combative approach to the establishment. Erskine put forward a revolutionary defence: that English law allowed for partial insanity; that is, it included recognition of people who suffered from bouts of periodic mental illness, but were otherwise well and able to function. Erskine suggested that Hadfield was such a person. Hadfield was diligent and rational when he was not in a religious frenzy; a supportive husband, who could also hold down a job, and to all intents and purposes professed to love the King. Erskine's success was such that the trial was unable to reach a proper conclusion. The case collapsed in rather confused circumstances, with Hadfield found not guilty, yet still remanded to Bethlem, while parliament regulated the judge-made outcome. The case resulted in the passing of the Criminal Lunatics Act 1800. This gave Hadfield a new status, while the law now had the power to detain him until 'His Majesty's pleasure be known', which for many years was the legal form for an indefinite sentence. Duly labelled as a criminal lunatic, and despite a brief escape from Newgate Prison, Hadfield remained a guest of His Majesty until his death in 1841.

The reform made a great difference. Now that the new sentence existed there came further Hadfields, all similarly afflicted and all requiring some form of secure accommodation. This point had been overlooked when the 1800 act was passed. There were precious few madhouses around England, and most of them were small establishments. As luck would have it, soon after Hadfield was tried, Bethlem decided that it had outgrown its old city space and needed larger premises. When the new hospital opened in St George's Fields in 1816, the government negotiated within it the first dedicated space for criminal lunatics. Two new wings were built on site, which became known as the State Criminal Lunatic Asylum. It was an opportunistic move rather than a long-term one, with much haggling before the deal was done and neither side was truly happy with the public-private partnership. Nor was there much capacity, for the extra wings had been squeezed into what were supposed to be the Bethlem grounds. When the state wings filled up a few decades later, more short-term space was purchased, first at Fisherton House Asylum in Salisbury and then as required, in ones and twos, at other outposts. As the national population mushroomed during the nineteenth century, so too did the small subset of criminal lunatics.

The Home Office, under Secretary Sir George Grey, decided in the late 1850s that this situation could not be allowed to continue. It sought a piece of land on which to build a dedicated special hospital. The site at Crowthorne that would become Broadmoor, part of the Crown estate of Windsor Forest, was chosen for being reasonably isolated, yet also easily accessible from London. Crowthorne village barely existed at the time, but Wellington College was being built nearby and was also due to gain a station on the London and South East Railway, so the area was ripe for development. The new asylum was to be perched high up on a ridge within the forest, commanding a magnificent, and suitably healthy view across the countryside below.

Plans were shelved briefly when the Whig government fell and Grey was removed from office, but after one of many parliamentary enquiries into lunacy the accelerator was pressed again. The Criminal Lunatic Asylums Act of 1860 allowed the government to act on its plan and fund construction of its own special asylum. Sir George Grey was back in his post by the time building had begun, and under his instruction the Home Office's prison architect, Sir Joshua Jebb, was given the task of designing the structure. Within three years an army of convicts had supplied forced labour; the woods had been cleared; several secure brick boxes reached up to the sky; Jebb was on his death bed; and Broadmoor was open for business.

* * *

For the first nine months of its existence, Broadmoor was a female-only hospital. This was for the very practical reason that the site design included fewer buildings on the female side, and they were finished first. There was a solitary female accommodation block, and it sat in an adjacent compound to the five male blocks that gestated slowly during the asylum's initial building phase. The plan was that once the five male blocks were ready, the remaining convict labour on site would retrench to what became Block 6, staying only to put the finishing touches to the other parts of the estate during the asylum's first winter. It was 27 February 1864 when the coaches of men from Bethlem and Fisherton began replicating the women's arrival. Patients like Edward Oxford and Richard Dadd were amongst those transferred.

By the end of 1864 there were 200 men to the 100 women present in the asylum. These numbers would swell further until there were around 500 patients in Victorian Broadmoor at any one time, in a ratio of roughly four men to every one woman. The patients came from all over England and Wales – as well as the military courts that spanned the British Empire – and across all social and educational divides. Broadmoor was generally a more representative institution than the county asylums, where the upper and middle-class mad might either be kept at home or sent off to a private house instead. Criminal law allowed for no such option, although of course there are caveats to that sweeping statement of inclusion. The mix of patients within the walls at Crowthorne varied continually from month to month and year to year over the duration of the Victorian period and anomalies still arose from the establishment prejudices of the judicial system. However, Broadmoor was a unique community and the statistics from the first year's intake of patients prove the varied flavour of its make up.

Most of the men could read and write, with around one in ten having enjoyed what was described as a 'superior' education. This contrasted with the female side, where only around a third could follow letters and no woman was considered educationally superior. This scholastic division between the sexes extended into the patients' backgrounds. It is true that on both sides by far the greater proportion of the patients came from labouring classes. More than half of the men either described themselves as labourers or had a manual occupation. On the female side it was extremely rare to find a woman who was not herself a worker or married to one. Within the wards were representatives of typical trades associated with female domestic drudgery – dressmakers, cleaners, hawkers and prostitutes.

The swell of labourers on the male side was joined by their obvious 'betters', like Richard Dadd the artist; a well-to-do surgeon and arsonist called George Houlton; four legal clerks; and another four commissioned officers in the armed forces. There was even William Ross Tuchet, the third son of the twentieth Baron Audley, known as 'the boy in the shed' to his family: the archetypal lunatic aristocrat, whose existence was hidden whenever the next edition of *Burke's* became due. The largely catatonic Tuchet and his fellow great and good sat side by side in the wards with the factory hands, tradesmen and rank and file soldiers, with whom they would have had fleeting contact in the world elsewhere.

Only half of the women were married, and perhaps there lies the reason for the lack of 'superior' well-educated women. The suggestion has been made that since the cause of many female admissions was an attack on their own children, the married middle-class Victorian lady was not likely to be found at Broadmoor. Any murderous tendencies such a lady might have had would have been deflected either by her distant relationship with her offspring or thwarted by the presence of the nanny or the governess. She would simply have had no opportunity to commit infanticide. Her husband was a different matter; in what was still a very patriarchal society, no one would dream of so interfering with the madness of the middle-class man.

The offences for which patients were admitted tended towards those involving direct physical harm. Around a quarter of the men and 40 per cent of the women were murderers; many others had attempted to kill. These patients, who had often dispatched their nearest and dearest, made up the bulk of the pleasure men and women who had been found not guilty but insane, in the manner of Hadfield. Otherwise, the average patient had probably been caught stealing and found guilty but then gone mad in jail. There was also the occasional fire starter amongst the pleasure men, as well as sex offenders, including paedophiles and those who had committed bestial acts. Then there were the traitorous, such as Edward Oxford and a small handful of Victorian men who had publicly wished the Queen ill. From these summits of harm the causes of admission sloped down to more gentle undulations of nuisance. Nineteenth century criminal law required a judge to pass the pleasure sentence for any defendant found innocent through insanity, with the result that relatively few patients ended up in Broadmoor for offences such as vagrancy, sending threatening letters or even attempting suicide.

One final observation might be made about the range of patients admitted. At the time of their initial interview with the medical staff, an attempt was made to categorise the lunatic. In Victorian terms this was the extent of diagnosis of the cause of a patient's insanity. Causes were pleasingly Victorian in their classification: the initial batch at Broadmoor included three masturbators (amongst them William Ross Tuchet), various sufferers of jealousy, grief or anxiety and even one poor soul who had been frightened into his present state. The catch-all code for such triggers was termed 'moral circumstances', and included such topics as: intemperance and vice; religious excitement; disappointment in love; and poverty. Yet, despite the Victorians' fondness for morality, a greater number of causes were attributed to physical conditions, even if these were not fully understood, such as fever, head injuries, and childbirth. With the majority of cases, the doctors did not even hazard a guess. Only around a third of the male cases and a little under half of the female ones were allocated some discernible genesis. For the rest, the prompt for their descent into insanity was unknown.

* * *

Two categories common to all the patients in Victorian Broadmoor were reflected in the name given to the asylum. One was legal and the other medical, and they were referred to by the epithets given to the patients: 'criminal' and 'lunatic'. Admission was granted only to those who satisfied both criteria, and it was this that made the institution a unique one.

The patients were all criminals due to their judicial history. Every patient had been arrested for a crime, charged by the magistrates and then dealt with by the courts. Most of the patients had been found 'not guilty by reason of insanity' (at least until 1883, when the standard form became 'guilty, but insane', in a vain hope that a denial of innocence would somehow deter lunatics from their criminal actions), just as James Hadfield had been in 1800. Usually this happened at their trial or at some point before it. Some patients did not even get as far as attending court to make a plea, while others were found insane on arraignment when they came to stand in the dock, but before any evidence was heard. Only if a case went to full hearing would the jury have been required to deliver a verdict of insanity based on the evidence put forward, usually by the defence. Whenever the call was made, the sentence was the same. These were the pleasure men and women, destined to remain in Crowthorne until what was now

Her Majesty's Pleasure was known. Although the balance varied, roughly two-thirds of the patient population at any time were 'pleasure'.

Complementing this group were the 'time' patients: criminals tried in court and found guilty. Sentence was passed in the usual manner and the accused removed as a convict to one of Her Majesty's prisons. Sentence length varied: most convicts at Broadmoor were serving somewhere between five and ten years; though their number included murderers who were serving a life sentence, commuted from their appointment with the gallows, as well as particularly difficult prisoners whose sentences could be measured in months. The usual passage into Broadmoor for the convict patient was that during their sentence they had become insane, and in need of treatment in an asylum. Those with lesser sentences and needs tended to be farmed out into the county asylum network, causing much angst in the provinces, with Broadmoor reserved only for the more truculent types.

The second, somewhat rarer, way in was reserved for capital offenders. If a convict faced the death penalty, then the Home Secretary might be petitioned to order a special inquiry into the condemned's sanity. A number of murderers were respited to Broadmoor's care in this way. Usually they retained the guilty verdict for their crime, like Mary Ann Parr, but very exceptionally they might become an innocent pleasure patient instead. This controversial option was the lifeline thrown to Christiana Edmunds. The existence of an escape route from the clutch of death (or even long-term incarceration) might beg the question of whether any fake lunatics were to be found within the walls at Crowthorne. Evidence suggests that Victorian Broadmoor did unwittingly house the occasional criminal who was shamming, though no one who might otherwise have met the noose. There are also indications that attempts to feign mental illness were often made without success. Broadmoor's staff were wise to the possibility of malingerers, and there was a revolving door that returned as many sane convicts to the prison system as it received. Quite apart from this, a sane convict soon discovered that sharing space with the lunatics was not necessarily preferable to the greater rationalities of jail.

For the lunatics were, by definition, insane. Though they were no longer thought of as being affected directly by the moon, they were affected by many things that did not so disturb other, non-lunatic people. There was still an element of the unknown about their disease, something intangible about how it moved from their minds to wreak havoc upon their bodies. The growth of alienists, or mind doctors, during the Victorian period was one manifestation of this curiosity. Far from progressing beyond the idea of lunacy, the alienists generally grappled with as many mysteries as they could imagine. It was only during the twentieth century that the word 'lunatic' ceased to be the industry norm, whereupon it rapidly became a somewhat guilty word, an incorrect way of describing a sufferer from mental illness. This seems a shame, and although it became a label and a source of stigma, perhaps the time is ripe for its reclaiming by those afflicted by the moon. It is a word of great power and potentially of empowerment. It could give status as much as imputation, for it still aptly conveys the loss of influence over one's actions to forces both outside our control and not fully understood.

Victorian definitions of types of insanity were rather different to our own, though they recognised many of the same phenomena. The starting point was the idea of 'moral' and 'physical' causes, something that would only begin to die out as the nineteenth century drew to a close. For the doctors at Broadmoor, each of these causes had then manifested themselves in a defined disease, which could be observed and a diagnosis inferred through the patient's habits, as well as through interview.

The principal diseases and diagnoses on offer to the Victorian physician are still recognisable today: mania; melancholia; dementia. Mania suggested an intensity of some extroverted, possibly violent, behaviour. Melancholia was its more introverted cousin, while dementia was a deterioration in some aspect of reason. Monomania was an obsession with a single subject; amentia, absence of mind, would now be described as learning disabilities, accepted now as something completely separate from mental illness. To these cognitive deficiencies, the Victorians added the concept of moral insanity, a disease free of delusions but where the mind was unable to think and behave as it should. Although it did not quite fit the modern term of psychopath, itself a rather overworked word, it is perhaps the nearest thing to it that the Victorians acknowledged.

Within that barrel of psychiatric apples, the first bobbing would have been undertaken by a patient's legal team. It was for counsel to show that the defendant's disease had led directly to the action of which they were accused and that consequently any *mens rea* (guilty state of mind, or culpability) was absent. Only then could a plea of insanity succeed.

In legal terms, the application of the medical principles were governed by case law. For many years, Hadfield's case provided a rudimentary precedent. The insanity defence was only refined in 1843 by what became known as the McNaughten Rules. Fittingly, this case involved another patient who spent time in both Bethlem and Broadmoor. Daniel McNaughten, a lathe worker from Glasgow, became convinced that he was being followed by spies in the control of Prime Minister Sir Robert Peel. He travelled down to London, almost certainly with the intention of killing Peel, but shot Peel's private secretary Edward Drummond instead. In the eyes of the popular press, McNaughten's crime was then compounded by the fact that he was found not guilty by reason of insanity. There was an outcry that no matter how mad McNaughten might be, it could never be mad enough for him not to get his criminal deserts. A House of Lords committee was forced to deliver guidance that confirmed the correctness of McNaughten's verdict.

The most quoted premise from the McNaughten case was that the defendant was unable to reason right from wrong, and so did not understand the nature or the quality of his or her actions. It was a fine judicial statement, at once precise and yet still leaving plenty of room for legal argument, and it allowed the Victorian lawyers increased scope. In practical terms, various approaches to insanity became popular with defence counsel. A history of hereditary insanity was considered to be a good bet, as was showing that your client suffered from delusions linked to some sort of traumatic event, past or present. A destitute man may believe his family to be better off in heaven, for example, or a new mother that her child was damned at birth and permanently blighted by sin. Similarly, the insane actor may be driven to his crime by an irresistible impulse, commanded by God or otherwise at the mercy of forces beyond his control. These forces might even be self-inflicted, as the Victorians believed that drink or religion, if taken to addictive levels, could effectively cauterise choice.

Broadmoor Hospital: By Way of Introduction

The casual observer might well conclude that the law was drawn for lunatics rather more generously than it is today. A modern alcoholic is unlikely to be found not guilty, and the perpetrator of crimes that we find it difficult to understand is no longer necessarily given any benefit of mental doubt. There are tests to complete these days, and analysis to be done. Yet many of the celebrated Victorian insanity cases concerned murder, and the law of the nineteenth century court had a heavier weight to balance on its scales of justice – that of the condemned's feet upon the gallows trapdoor. Perhaps the law is only human, after all.

* * *

Once a defendant had been judged as not culpable for their actions due to their mental health, they moved from being criminals to becoming criminal lunatics. The pleasure sentence was invoked. For the convicts, this judgement came initially from a prison doctor rather than a jury. In both situations, the Home Secretary was obliged effectively to agree to the decision and therefore give it the seal of approval. Only then would a patient be transferred to Broadmoor to begin their 'moral treatment'.

As mentioned earlier, the routine of patient life was not just an integral part of care, it was often the only part. It began as soon as a patient was assigned to one of the blocks. Each block at Broadmoor was quite separate, and therefore segregated from the others. On the female side, one initial block housed all the patients for the first few years. There was a subdivide between its three wards: one ward for the more aggressive or noisy patients; one ward for those who were low risk; and one ward for those in-between. When the second block was opened in 1867, the more aggressive women were siphoned off into that and female Block 1 became the passive block.

On the male side, Block 1 was one of the 'back' or 'refractory' blocks and was joined by Block 6 in 1868. These two blocks were the male accommodation for violent and destructive types. The name 'back blocks' came from their position on the north side of the site, without direct access to the beautiful views of trees and fields which could be enjoyed across the southern terrace. All blocks had a separate airing court, but most had a door that took you to the terrace for a walk above the landscape of the Blackwater

Valley. In contrast, the men of the back blocks had bricked-in airing courts and were hidden from the rest of the site, cut off from a spiritually uplifting view and with only the sky visible to them. 'Limited, cheerless and wet' is how the Government's Commissioners in Lunacy described them on one visit. Eventually a first floor day room was constructed, so back block patients could at least glimpse a view from inside the blocks, but the two buildings remained a secure area within a secure area, such was the nature of their clientèle. The attendants who walked the galleries of the back blocks had uniforms with hidden buttons and equipped with padding, and a patient's room was likely to hold bedding only, probably not even a bed frame.

The direct opposite of the back blocks were those immediately to their south, which were Blocks 2 and 5 respectively. Patients in these blocks were considered the lowest risk, and enjoyed greater access around the site: their airing courts led directly on to the terrace, and they were more likely to be granted membership of the walking parties that perambulated around the wider estate. Block 2 in particular became known as the 'privilege block', where patients had the most freedom to plan their days. Their insanity did not affect their daily lives and they could also be trusted to spend their time fruitfully at work, in their rooms, in the communal rooms in their block, or watching the world go by on the terrace. Block 2 was where VIPs and the press were brought if a bit of Victorian public relations work was required. Oxford, Dadd and Minor were all sometime residents of Block 2.

Block 3 housed the infirmary, and Block 4 included the admissions ward, where all the men made their first entrance, but both these blocks also housed those in-between patients who did not fit consistently into the categories of being either dangerous or placid. These two were the biggest blocks, both housing 100 patients, and formed one aisle each off the main administration block of the hospital. As a result, Blocks 3 and 4 have gained listed status, while the other blocks have not.

This total capacity proved sufficient for the women, but not for the men. In 1887, Block 1 was joined to Block 2, and Block 5 joined to Block 6 to accommodate an extra 70 patients, transferred from the prison system. That particular solution lasted for around ten years, before Block 7 was formulated at the end of the Victorian period

Broadmoor Hospital: By Way of Introduction

and eventually opened in 1902. Its existence led to a piece of asylum humour, as the Broadmoor Cemetery became known as Block 8.

When Broadmoor opened, each block offered a mix of single rooms and dormitories sleeping eight patients. The idea was that patients would sleep in dormitories unless there seemed a good reason for them not to; either because it was not safe to have them in a communal space or because their health might be improved by having their own room. In practice, single rooms were found to be preferable and the number of dormitories was gradually reduced throughout the period.

The result was that the typical Victorian patient had a single room to themselves, measuring 12 feet long by 8 feet wide. Most rooms came equipped with a single horsehair mattress, a bedstead and a desk. The linen was changed twice a week, and both sheets and blankets were available. Patients were also allowed personal possessions in their room if it was safe to have them, though inevitably what was considered safe varied from ward to ward and block to block. A set of cufflinks proudly worn in Block 2 might become a potential weapon in Block 1; a belt or braces might offer self-esteem to one patient, but a method of suicide to another.

Once assigned to a block, a patient could settle into his or her version of the moral treatment routine. For most of the hospital's early decades, that would mean the day starting at six o'clock (or seven in the winter), when the day shift attendants came on duty and the chaplain started prayers, and ending at seven o'clock in the evening, when the night shift came on. In between those fixed hours, the day was punctuated by segments of time filled by meals, work and leisure. Groups of patients moved *en masse*, like shoals of fish.

The bulk of the day would be spent at work, if a patient was able to perform a labouring task. For those blessed with only basic skills, work consisted principally of ward cleaning; the endless washing, scrubbing and polishing required to keep the asylum spotless. For the more able, a range of skilled occupations were available, all consistent with the self-sufficient approach to Victorian asylum life. Able women were employed as seamstresses or in the laundry; able men as tailors, shoemakers, upholsterers, tinsmiths or carpenters, as well as on the asylum farm, garden or wider estate where they could tend crops in the fields. Every piece of underwear or shoe leather stitched, every chair covered or table jointed went into the asylum stores or buildings. The patients stocked Broadmoor and benefited directly their quality of life.

Such leisure time as there was might be spent reading or playing board games in the day rooms or in the summer, playing outdoor sports, such as croquet and cricket. Walking was encouraged: either in the airing court attached to the block or, for the more trusted patients, strolling (accompanied, of course) around the local area. In time, carriage drives also became an option for the well-behaved lady patients.

Special interests were encouraged, such as Dadd's painting or Minor's research work. A number of patients took to painting or model-building or learning to play musical instruments. Many patients also wrote, either contentedly to family and friends, or discontentedly to others, recording either their own unhappy state or agitating the staff or persons in authority to do something about it.

This more creative side to asylum life sometimes sought outlet through its entertainment programme. From very early on, male patients were encouraged to join in with concerts and the occasional dramatic presentation – mostly humorous – while female patients were allowed to hold a fortnightly dance. Soon, an asylum brass band had been formed from amongst the staff and patients and played regularly at all these events.

As time went on, the concept of evening entertainment was developed. A regular troupe of staff, and sometimes patients, would tread the boards above the footlights of the central hall. Shows included such turns as Medical Superintendent David Nicolson hamming it up in *HMS Pinafore* or Steward Charles Phelps and his daughter Florence playing a duet on piano and violin. Nicolson even formed a choral society to further the influence of light operetta. Most bizarrely, the handful of ethnic minority patients were treated to the occasional extreme make-up of a minstrel group known as 'The Broadmoor Blacks'. Amateur dramatics and musical appreciation thrived. If a production was particularly fine, then the local village families and their children were invited in to watch, on payment of a small admission fee. These public shows were used to raise money for good causes, such as other patient pursuits or for the local church. Souvenir programmes were produced by one of the patients, a teacher, who had developed a talent with the printing press.

Very occasionally, an external artiste was invited to put on a performance. These tended to be music hall variety acts that would augment the asylum's own repertoire: magicians and illusionists or demonstrators of feats of memory. They were always men. The most interesting visitor by far was John Williams Benn, then a publisher, but also a part-time painter of portraits while blindfold. Benn went on to become an important politician: chair of London County Council, a member of parliament, a baronet and grandfather to Tony Benn. His involvement with Broadmoor came about through his brother, William Rutherford Benn, who had killed their father in 1883.

Family and friends were considered to be an important part of every patient's life. In true authoritarian fashion, a judgement was made as to whether the relationship was harmful or beneficial to a patient's well-being. Letters might be withheld, either on the way out or the way in, and incoming correspondence containing bad news tended to be delivered in person. Visits were encouraged, and a visitor had only to write to the medical superintendent and arrange a date on which they might call. In practice, for many friends or family visiting was restricted by its financial impact. Time spent not working was time spent not earning, quite apart from the costs of train and other transport. The asylum carriage was often prepared to pick up guests from the local railway stations, and accommodation was provided at reasonable rates by hostelries nearby, yet a visit was still a luxury that many patients with far-flung families never received.

The isolated life of the Victorian lunatic is something that we might struggle to imagine. Similarly, the lack of physical comfort, the cold and the dark. When Broadmoor first opened, there was no heating in any of the bedrooms and only open fires and hot air grates in the day rooms provided any warmth. During the 1880s central heating was introduced slowly throughout the blocks, powered first by solid fuel and then by gas. The men continued to receive some relief through the hot air system, which was finally omnipresent in 1889; the women had the luxury of radiators a few years earlier. Before this, even if you had wished to stay up in your bedroom at night the grinding cold would encourage you to get underneath the covers. But then, staying up was hardly practicable. With no artificial lighting in the patients' bedrooms, once the sun went down all became black. In the winter months, patients spent half the day in darkness. Oil and gas lamps were used only for lighting the communal rooms and corridors. In the bedrooms only the moon, a lunatic's true companion, provided any respite from the gloom.

Sanitary conditions were also rudimentary. For many years the asylum staff harboured dark suspicions about the desirability of water closets, and it was only during the building alterations of the 1880s that flushing mechanisms were finally seized more enthusiastically. Earth closets were the order of the day for the first two decades of Broadmoor's existence. The clearing of the closets was another part of the daily routine, and probably one for strong stomachs. Running water was available for washing, and patients were washed daily and bathed once a week in the ward bathroom. A toothbrush and comb were available to anyone 'capable of appreciating their use'. Male patients were also shaved regularly by an attendant, if they wished to be. Such was the risk attached to this operation that, while one attendant worked the razor, another attendant was always present to keep an eye on proceedings.

What the patients lacked in environmental comforts was compensated for by clothing. Male patients were granted one nightshirt a week and two day shirts, worn alternatively over a flannel vest. Strong grey trousers and a darker jacket of the same colour were the usual over-garments. The clothing on the women's side showed a little more variation, though patients did not enjoy the sometimes jaunty patterns afforded to the women of other public asylums. Sobriety was the watchword, with a gingham check the only nod to levity. On both sides in the privilege blocks patients could also be found wearing their own clothes, which was part of the humanising process that might prepare a recovering patient for discharge.

The final aspect to patient routine was food. A working patient would receive four meals a day, while the idle and the infirm found that lunch bypassed them. Wherever they were on the estate, everyone returned to their block to be fed, as each block had its own dining room. There was a little ballet performed at the commencement and conclusion of every meal: each item of

Broadmoor Hospital: By Way of Introduction

cutlery was removed from the block's canteen and counted out by an attendant, before being counted back and returned again when dining was complete. Grace was said before and after the meal. Although the patient diet varied within the Victorian period, and also seasonally, depending on what food was available, it is possible to describe a basic pattern of victuals on offer. For breakfast, patients generally had tea and bread and butter. Lunch, provided for the workers, was usually bread and cheese. In the late afternoon a typical tea would be mutton, beef or pork with potatoes (or vegetables if in season), followed by a steamed pudding. The final meal was supper, a further helping of bread and butter with tea.

Patients drank primarily tea and a very weak beer. Three-quarters of a pint of this beer might be given with the evening meal, almost certainly on the basis that it contained a little extra nourishment. Beer was commonplace in Victorian asylums, and at Broadmoor further rations of it were usually given to workers during the day. Its alcoholic content was so low as to be negligible and its description as ale is flattering. However, strong liquor did have its place on the medicine shelf: brandy or other fortified drinks might be offered to patients who were sick and suffering from physical debility.

On very special occasions, all thoughts of routine were jettisoned and celebration was had, as in any village throughout the country. Christmas was always marked with a special meal, and as a New Year treat the women were also able to dress up for an annual ball, at which the male doctors and other senior staff would take turns to dance with the patients in their care. National festivities were also part of the calendar: on 21 June 1887 the patients were all treated to a lunch in honour of Queen Victoria's Golden Jubilee. Roast beef and plum pudding was served, and afterwards dried fruits and tobacco were dispensed. How this was received by those few patients who had designs on the Queen's head is not recorded.

* * *

Charged with implementing the routine was a staff of around 100 asylum employees. Like the patients, the Broadmoor employees ranged across the social spectrum and in many ways, their make up also resembled any English village. At the top of the feudal order was the Lord of the Manor, the medical superintendent, who with his physician subordinates formed the first family of the estate. The next layer in the village pyramid was of management: each block had a principal attendant to manage the nursing care; there was a steward to run the stores and grounds; a clerk to attend to estate business; and a matron to look after the female side. In turn, these members of staff looked after those who formed the base of the pyramid, such as the gardeners, the cooks, the boiler stokers and gatekeepers, as well as the massed ranks of attendants who made up the bulk of the establishment. The community's spiritual needs were administered by the chaplain, who was effectively the parish priest.

Of the characters who made up this team, two men were there at the start: Medical Superintendent John Meyer and his deputy, William Orange. They were the first appointments made by the Council of Supervision that was created by the Home Office to oversee the new Criminal Lunatic Asylum. Both men came from the Surrey Asylum in Wandsworth. Meyer had an imperial background: he had served as a surgeon in the Crimea and then run an asylum in Tasmania before returning to England. He was nearly 50 when he assumed command of Broadmoor. Orange, in contrast, was a generation younger and had no military interests. The son of a dissenting preacher, he had acquired a strong tendency to question the orthodox. He was an atheist and an academic, and combined his work as Meyer's deputy with study for a doctorate at the University of Heidelberg.

These two men set about recruiting the rest of the original staff, including a third doctor who completed the entire medical team charged with the responsibility for Her Majesty's lunatics. It was an incredible level of work to entrust to just three people, and reflected the paucity of interventions available to them. A large part of their clinical work was observational, and they juggled their time between clinical and management decisions. The medical superintendent in particular was expected to fulfil the roles of chief executive and head of personnel, as well as that of senior doctor, and he expected his fellow professionals to assist him as much as they could. The result was that each man had notionally around 150 patients under their control, though in practice the junior doctor – the assistant medical officer – was assigned the greater share. Usually either the super or the deputy took on the women, while the chaplain doubled up his role as spiritual leader with a responsibility for patient education and other forms of self-improvement.

The attendants who formed the nursing staff often had no previous medical background, and physical presence was considered as important an attribute as any other. Many of the male staff had either served in the forces or come from the prison service to join Broadmoor. The early years, in particular, saw a mixed success rate with this recruitment strategy. Familiarity with a regimented life did not necessarily make for a happy attendant. During the asylum's first decade the turnover rate for attendants approached 50 per cent annually. This can partly be explained by the fact that female attendants in Victorian times (and for many decades thereafter) were expected to resign their position upon marriage, but discipline among the ranks was also a significant problem. Within the asylum archive is a series of 'defaulters' books' that list dishonesty, dormancy, incompetence, tardiness and drunkenness amongst the attendants' many sins.

It would be wrong though, to conclude that this was an inhumane regime where brutality and immorality were commonplace. On the contrary, there were a number of rules in place that provided attendants with a moral compass and which emphasised the compassionate attitude they should strive for. 'Kindness and forbearance are first principles in the care and management of persons of unsound mind; few such persons are beyond their influence. The mischievous will become somewhat less troublesome, the dirty less careless; the irritable and violent often render most essential service to the attendants who treat them firmly, justly, and kindly,' ran the opening paragraph of the attendants' instruction manual.

Physical restraint was seen as a last resort and all incidents tended to be noted in one record or another. In general, any restraint used was an immediate response to a potentially dangerous situation, rather than a calculated act of control. The only Broadmoor medic who countenanced the use of straitjackets was Meyer, and even he used it sparingly. Everyone else considered it beyond the pale.

It is possible to cast Meyer – a squat, prosperous man with swept over hair and a wavy, reddish beard – in the role of Broadmoor's heartless overlord. He was a man who seems to have fought with most of his senior staff at one time or another, even Orange; a man who had the most violent male patients segregated in caged areas of their blocks; a man who perhaps was not the most enlightened brain doctor of the Victorian age. A rapid decrease in the turnover of attendants followed Meyer's passing. Perhaps Meyer's experiences of war or colonial convicts had made him battle-hardened, uncommunicative and distant, but nevertheless he also had the unenviable task of trying to find a blueprint for a new type of institution, as well as dealing with the inevitable flaws in the design and fabric of the building he inherited. He also suffered from ill health. After he was attacked by a patient called John Hughes in the asylum chapel in March 1866 and struck a severe blow on the temple by a large stone, he never fully recovered. Hughes was a despoiler of royal portraits hung within the holy confines of a north London church. He stated that Meyer had accused him of 'murdering the Queen of Heaven' during a previous conversation and that he had felt obliged to avenge that insult. Meyer was put on the sick list and Hughes was put in solitary confinement.

Attacks would form a part of each of the first three medical superintendents' careers, and were an occupational hazard for all the staff. Orange, who became Meyer's successor, was assaulted in 1882 by an insane cleric called Henry Dodwell, who argued that trying to kill the superintendent was the only way to draw attention to his wrongful detention. Dodwell's argument was an extension of the one that he had used a few years before, when he shot at the Master of the Rolls to draw attention to the injustices of a legal action that he was pursuing. Orange's deputy, David Nicolson, was similarly attacked by a chair maker called Henry Forrester in 1884. Nicolson was well enough to return to work and take promotion in due course, though he was also the only superintendent to suffer two attacks. James Lyons, a convict patient, went on to throw a stone at his head in 1889. Despite these twin assaults, Nicolson might still consider himself more fortunate than the deputy he had succeeded. William Douglas lasted four

Broadmoor Hospital: By Way of Introduction

months at Broadmoor in 1871 before being injured so badly that he never returned to work.

The personality of the Broadmoor medical staff was bound to leave an impression on the institution that they ran. So it was that when Meyer died suddenly in Exeter in May 1870, while returning from a visit to his dying brother-in-law, his 37-year-old assistant began immediately to change the culture of the organisation that he had acquired. William Orange spent 16 years in charge of Broadmoor, and these years had a profound effect on the asylum. The cultural chord that he sounded, echoes of which still resound today, can be summed up by the twin pillars of rehabilitation and public protection that Orange's Broadmoor represented.

Orange's Broadmoor was one in which arts, crafts and sports flourished. Patients were integrated as much as possible and social interaction encouraged. They were rewarded financially for their work and encouraged to spend their money responsibly. At the same time, Orange took a paternalistic approach to deciding whether or not his charges were well enough to resume life outside the walls. Only if he was absolutely sure that they would not reoffend and had a suitably safe home life would an invitation be made to petition the Home Office.

Many of Orange's patients have left behind testimony of the genuine warmth they felt for him. Barring the occasional patient who considered Orange to be part of the infernal conspiracy concocted against them, most residents wrote respectfully and kindly to him. To a certain extent this might be expected of a man who held the keys to their futures, but the emotions seem to run deeper than that. Two things might serve to illustrate this: that Orange received a number of spontaneous letters of goodwill after Dodwell's attack on him; and that the man who assaulted poor Dr Douglas was one of several patients who felt able to write asking Orange for a little money many years after discharge. Orange usually obliged his ex-charges with a small sum to tide them over, and there is no reason to suppose that Leest was an exception.

The staff enjoyed life under Orange too. He improved their terms and conditions, as well as making Broadmoor a happier place to be. Orange did not enjoy the same, spiky relationship that Meyer had with his underlings, and he may also have lent a different touch to recruitment. Care was the new imperative, and that included care for one's own team. Nicolson's only recorded criticism of his boss was for his micro-management, feeling that at times Orange's attention to detail risked missing the wood for the trees.

Orange was severely incapacitated after Dodwell's attack and spent long periods of time absent from work through sickness. The result was that from the summer of 1882 David Nicolson gradually assumed more control of Broadmoor, and an additional medical officer was appointed to help cover for the temporary losses of the medical superintendent. When Orange finally retired in 1886 it was Nicolson who took over, a Scot who had previously been at Portsmouth Prison before joining Broadmoor in 1876. Nicolson provided continuity, as well as a more strategic approach than Orange. He was just as caring, but perhaps a rather better manager. Orange was awarded the Order of the Bath for his services and later returned to the asylum as a member of the Council of Supervision.

In that any long-running institution bears a received memory and received values from those who have trod its corridors along the years, I feel the modern hospital still owes a debt to Orange and to Nicolson. Nevertheless, although my impression of their years at the helm is one of great success in their enterprise, when the time came for Nicolson to retire in 1895, his deputy was not selected to succeed him. For the first time in Broadmoor's history, a break was made. The doctor in question, John Baldwin Isaac, was as old as Nicolson and not quite the high-flyer that his bosses had been. He had been at Broadmoor even longer than Nicolson had.

Instead, the post was given to the suitably-named Richard Brayn, who became the last of the Victorian superintendents. Like Nicolson, Brayn came from the prison service, but there the similarities ended. Brayn was a great believer in running a tight, punitive ship, which occasionally put him in conflict with other professionals around him. He found seclusion – the asylum euphemism for solitary confinement – to be a very agreeable method of control and used it willingly. The result was that the asylum's pillar of rehabilitation was perhaps slightly more neglected than the pillar of public protection during Brayn's time in charge, although the positives in the lopsided edifice were a lack of successful escapes, coupled with Brayn's success in becoming the first superintendent not to suffer personal injury. The boot camp approach also saw benefits in spit and polish: Brayn embarked on a wide-ranging programme of painting and decorating, which cheered up many of the tired hospital interiors.

Broadmoor ended the Victorian era with an updated and more personable version of Meyer still in charge. Brayn was a competent leader and well-respected by his peers, even if perhaps the same affection for Orange and Nicolson did not extend to him. That he was appreciated more outside Broadmoor's walls was confirmed when his retirement was followed by the knighthood denied to Nicolson.

* * *

By the time that Queen Victoria finally relinquished her grip on the British throne, Broadmoor had become a recognised part of the medical, judicial and social landscape of England and Wales. It was a much bigger place than it had been in 1863, though its patient base and the wide range of needs it catered for remained roughly the same as when it had opened. So too were the treatments for criminal lunatics still rooted in the nineteenth century rather than the more fanciful ideas developing in mental health care. There was no *fin de siècle* feel about the place: the Victorian asylum lived on.

Some of what remained of the Victorian asylum in 1901 still remains today; not just the bricks and mortar, but the records from that time, which allow us to glimpse behind the walls and try to better understand what we mean by Broadmoor. A handful of these records have been used to draw together the stories that follow, though there are so many to choose from that providing a representative picture of the place may well remain outside my reach.

One of the incredible features of the Broadmoor archive is that there is something for everyone. Whatever your interest, whatever your angle, the stories are true, the people are real, and the history is there to be discovered. You may wish to have your prejudices challenged or reinforced; to have your expectations met, dashed or confounded. Whatever reason you have come for, please do enjoy your tour round Victorian Broadmoor.

2

Edward Oxford: Shooting at Royalty

Many Victorian lunatics were only too aware of their Queen and Empress. As the national figure of authority, she fulfilled a key place in many a delusion. Every county asylum was likely to include patients who felt, rightly or wrongly, that they had their own direct line to the monarchy, and occasionally these patients had come close enough to Victoria to worry the local magistrates. In these cases the law on criminal lunacy would swing into action.

The county set of patients tended to be those who were considered to be no real threat to the sovereign's fair head. They may well have uncovered some dangerous conspiracy and been sent by God to warn the Queen of it; or perhaps they had been delivered of a fierce desire to marry one of Victoria's many offspring. Some of these messengers came quietly upon having their collars felt, while others committed a public order offence and received a short prison sentence at one of the lower courts. At some point, these lunatics were transferred quietly to their local hospital and left to pursue Her Majesty from a safer distance.

Broadmoor's role in managing this type of behaviour was wholly linked to the preservation of the Queen from serious harm. The patients it received after royal encounters were high profile and the subject of media frenzy. These patients were not brought before the bench on trivial offences, but on a charge of high treason. Edward Oxford was the first.

Edward Oxford: Shooting at Royalty

Edward Oxford was born in Birmingham on 9 April 1822, the third of seven children to Edward senior and Hannah Oxford. At his trial, Hannah outlined an abusive marriage to a violent and bewildering man, a goldsmith who would threaten her with violence and jump around 'like a baboon'. His own father, Oxford's grandfather, was allegedly an alcoholic and an absentee seaman. Hannah and Edward senior split not long before the latter died, when Oxford was seven. The date of death was 10 June 1829, a date that may well have imprinted itself on the young Edward's memory.

Oxford grew up in both Birmingham and Lambeth, sometimes with his mother for company or members of his extended family, sometimes boarded out at school alone. It was a peripatetic, if supported existence. His mother was always able to find work, and the two of them remained close despite the economic necessity of their occasional parting. However, Oxford's mother would later testify that she was already worried about him. He had 'eccentricities', which included a fondness for inappropriate giggling fits and playing about with sticks and gunpowder.

Hannah Oxford's family were publicans, and so after Oxford completed his schooling he took bar work, first from his aunt in Hounslow and then later at various establishments in central London. Oxford was a pale youth with brown eyes and auburn hair, around five foot six inches tall. Instead of socialising he was happier to be reading at home, something that was of less interest to the Victorian courtroom, but which has been observed as relevant by subsequent investigators. For Oxford liked the sensational, and he absorbed his library's fantasy world into his own. He began to write.

Oxford created a fictitious military society called Young England. Members were to be armed with a brace of pistols, a sword, a rifle and a dagger. There was a uniform too, and the red bows on Oxford's cap highlighted him as a captain of this society, able to command a hundred men. On paper at least there were another 400 members who had all signed up to a manifesto drafted by 'A W Smith' the Young England secretary. In reality, not only was Oxford the sole member of Young England but he had also begun to generate activity on the imaginary members' behalf. He created incidents in which his society had taken part and detailed the subterfuge required of a terrorist organisation. He wrote letters to himself from fictional correspondents, commending his own heroism. Oxford was no longer living his own life; he was acting it out in the third person.

In the spring of 1840, Oxford could be found in London working as a pot boy or barman at The Hog in the Pound, along Oxford Street, and living with his mother and sister in lodgings in Camberwell. It was the latest in a succession of short-term posts, and it was not going well. The giggling fits had become more frequent. Oxford's guffaws as the landlord's wife fell down the storeroom stairs spelt the end of this latest employment. At the beginning of May 1840, Oxford left The Hog in the Pound without further work to go to.

A week after he quit his job, his mother left Camberwell for a regular trip to Birmingham to visit relatives, and Oxford was left largely to his own devices. It seems reasonable to assume that during this period Oxford's separation between fantasy and reality became hopelessly blurred. Meanwhile, he decided to buy some pistols. Five weeks later, on the late spring evening of 10 June 1840 – 11 years to the day after his father's death – he took up a position on a footpath at Constitution Hill, near Buckingham Palace. He waited for the young Queen Victoria and Prince Albert to be driven out from the palace in an open carriage, and when they drew level with him, he fired theatrically two shots in succession from separate pistols at the Queen. She was four months pregnant at the time with her first child, Victoria, the Princess Royal.

Immediately, various members of the public seized Oxford and disarmed him. He put no effort into getting away and was quite open about what he had done, exclaiming "It was I, it was me that did it." What was not clear was exactly what he had done, as he had certainly fired two pistols at their Majesties, but whether those pistols could have harmed anyone would never be resolved. No bullets were ever found, and despite Oxford's initial contention that the pistols were loaded, the Crown was unable to prove in court that they were armed when Oxford discharged them. For the rest of his life, Oxford always maintained that the pistols contained only gunpowder.

Oxford was arrested and the decision was made to charge him with treason. His lodgings were searched and a box found containing the intricate rules of Young England. His mother was retrieved from Birmingham and interviewed by the Metropolitan Police. Oxford himself was put up before the Cabinet and subjected to interrogation by the great and good of government. It must have been an experience to rival any that he had read about in his books.

Inevitably, his custody attracted much attention, with even an employee from Madame Tussaud's making the trek to Newgate to gain an impression of Oxford's face. As a result, it was decided to postpone his trial until every possible enquiry had been made into both his background and his possible motives. Initially, there had been concern that Young England was real and preparing to strike at the heart of English life, so it was vital for the establishment to lay that lie to rest. Oxford's behaviour in custody gave a truer picture. He was manic – either elated or sobbing – and it was relatively straightforward to decide that insanity would be used as his defence.

On Monday 6 July 1840, the Old Bailey was packed with citizens fortunate enough to have obtained a ticket for admission to the trial. Oxford appeared largely oblivious to proceedings, even though his life was technically at issue. He sat and daydreamed while the prosecution presented a large amount of eyewitness evidence for the night in question. Then various family members and friends testified that Oxford had always seemed of unsound mind, quite apart from the fact that both his grandfather and father had exhibited signs of mental illness and were alcoholics. These points were important to the Victorians, for whom both drink and hereditary influence were strong causal factors for insanity. Hannah Oxford recounted the sorry tale of her former husband's domestic violence and intimidating behaviour, as well as Edward's own peculiar habits and obsessions.

The principal medical witnesses had examined Oxford in Newgate, and now they presented their conclusions. Dr Thomas Hodgkin considered that Oxford had a 'lesion of the will' and Dr John Conolly, Head of the Hanwell Lunatic Asylum, believed that Oxford had suffered a disease of the brain, evidenced by the shape of his head. Conolly had asked Oxford why he shot at the Queen, and Oxford replied "Oh, I may as well shoot at her as anybody else". The defence called other medics too: Dr William

Dingle Chowne agreed that Oxford could not control his impulses; while Dr James Fernandez Clarke thought Oxford was a hysterical imbecile. All agreed that Oxford was of unsound mind.

These were significant names in Victorian medicine. Conolly was the man who had destroyed every form of restraint used at Hanwell and promoted the new 'moral' regime of mental health care through routine and responsibility that would become the staple treatment in the asylum system. Clarke was an acclaimed medical author and a major contributor to *The Lancet*, while Hodgkin was an eminent pathologist who gave his name to Hodgkin's disease, and Chowne was a respected manager at Charing Cross Hospital and a leading advocate of sanitary reform.

The next day, the jury returned to acquit Oxford on the grounds of insanity. He received the sentence of all such lunatics since Hadfield's case. He was to be detained until Her Majesty's pleasure be known, and considering Her Majesty was his target, her pleasure was unlikely to be known soon.

Within a fortnight, Oxford was removed to the State Criminal Lunatic Asylum at Bethlem, then in Southwark, to begin his sentence. The experience seems to have given him some form of shock cure. Here was an eccentric boy of 18 shut away on a ward populated by both chronic and acute cases of mental illness, some exhibiting regular displays of violence. There was not the segregation that would be later found at Broadmoor.

There are comparatively few records from Oxford's time at Bethlem, though some notes from London were copied up into his Broadmoor case notes and give a flavour of what his new life was like. An entry for 16 February 1854 stated that: 'No note has ever been made of this case, and no record kept of the state of his mind at the time of his admission, but from the statements of the attendants and those associated with him he appears to have conducted himself with great propriety at all times'. Indeed, Oxford seems to have become a model patient at Bethlem, industrious and studious. He spent much time drawing, reading and in study; learning French, German and Italian to a standard of virtual fluency, while obtaining some knowledge of Spanish, Greek and Latin, as well as practising the violin. The Bethlem doctors also reported that he could play draughts and chess better than any other patient. He became a painter and decorator on the wards, and was gainfully employed within the hospital. Of his crime, the notes observed that 'He now laments the act which probably originated in a feeling of excess vanity and a desire to become notorious if he could not be celebrated'. Celebrity had been his undoing.

Presumably Oxford's positive influence on the ward was missed by the Bethlem authorities when he was moved to Broadmoor ten years later, even if the London hospital was generally glad to be rid of the criminal class. It was 30 April 1864, and Oxford had just celebrated his forty-second birthday. His health on arrival in Crowthorne was stated to be good, though it was noted that he suffered from constipation (always a worry for Victorian healthcare) and some swelling in his lower legs. Twenty-four years had passed since that performance on Constitution Hill and Oxford was an altogether different person from the callow youth who had acted out his fiction.

His notes on arrival in Broadmoor record: 'A well conducted industrious man apparently sane, has been rather out of health since last Christmas and has suffered from urethritis since his admission here – this he attributes to his having taken various unusual things to drink just before leaving Bethlem. He is now in better general health. He states that he fired a pistol charged with powder only at the Queen on 10 June 1840. That he did it under the impression that he should thereby become a noted person and that he had not the smallest intention of injuring Her Majesty'.

Oxford carried on at Broadmoor with the diligent application to hard work seen at Bethlem, labouring daily as a wood grainer and a painter and being very well-behaved. Indeed, it was increasingly obvious not only that Oxford no longer posed a risk to anyone, but also that he was completely sane. In such a case, the new Criminal Lunatic Asylum had a duty to report it. Sir William Hayter, the Chair of Broadmoor's scrutiny body, the Council of Supervision, wrote to Home Secretary Sir George Grey in November 1864 stating his belief that Oxford was of sound mind. Not only did John Meyer, Broadmoor's Medical Superintendent, testify to this, but also Charles Hood, who served as another member of the Council and had been Oxford's previous physician at Bethlem. Hood reported that Oxford had been sane since at least 1854, when the patient was first in his care. Neither did Oxford neglect to show appropriate remorse to the Queen: Hood wrote that he wished to 'endeavour to remove from the memory of his benefactor the sin of the past by a steady and pure life for the future'. Hayter concluded with the suggestion that Oxford was perfectly capable of being allowed to make his own way in the world.

Nevertheless, Oxford's case could not be divorced so easily from its political dimension. Grey ignored Hayter's request. He had been Judge Advocate General in the government in 1840, and perhaps he was uncomfortable with allowing the discharge of a case in which he probably had an interest. As a result, Oxford stayed on in the asylum until September 1867, when new Home Secretary Gathorne Hardy was prepared to look at the case again. Hardy asked Hayter to provide an up-to-date report on Oxford's mental condition. Subsequently, Oxford was offered discharge on the condition that he went overseas to one of the colonies, and never returned to the United Kingdom. Oxford was willing to accept the terms and Meyer proposed that he arrange a passage for his patient to Australia. Oxford himself had suggested that he be delivered to Melbourne. This may well have been inspired by his own closeness to George Haydon, one time Steward of Bethlem and friend to many of its long-term patients. Haydon had spent much time in Australia as a young man and had a strong affection for the country. Melbourne had also been his first port of call. Haydon was also in contact with Broadmoor as well as Oxford, and Meyer was happy to take his advice. There seemed little point in Oxford going somewhere that he would be unhappy, and any enthusiasm for his destination would have been seen as beneficial for his mental health.

Various practicalities required attention before Oxford could leave. Firstly, the patient was visited by 12 officers from the Metropolitan Police, who took notes about his appearance and photographed him, should he attempt to return to Albion's shores. Sadly, no copy of the photograph survives in the Broadmoor archives. Secondly, it was made clear to Oxford that if he ever set foot again in the British Isles, he would be locked up for good. Thirdly, he needed to be readied for his new adventure. Through Haydon, over £43 was deposited in Oxford's personal cash account. Twenty-five pounds went to pay his passage, while a trip to Heelas's department store in Reading and a gentleman's outfitter took three more for clothing and other essentials. This left the grand total of £22 10s, when added to his existing balance, which was given to Oxford in cash to help him get started in his new life.

The warrant for Oxford's discharge arrived at Broadmoor towards the end of October, and his passage, booked in the name of John Freeman, was arranged for a month later. Accompanied by Charles Phelps, the Steward at Broadmoor, Oxford travelled to Plymouth on 26 November 1867. The next day he boarded HMS *Suffolk*, bound for Melbourne. He and Phelps waited patiently on board for several days as the ship was detained in port, until she finally set sail on 3 December. Phelps was made to sign an affidavit that 'To the best of my knowledge and belief Oxford was on board when she sailed'.

Phelps could be relied upon. Oxford certainly sailed to Australia and he went on to make something rather special of his life there. This is not reflected in the Broadmoor archive, where the only subsequent, and inaccurate intelligence about Oxford came from a letter from Haydon to Dr Nicolson in 1883. Haydon quoted an article from *The Age*, a Melbourne newspaper, of which he had been made aware. The article, included with the letter, was about a man called John Oxford and was dated 4 May 1880. It stated that John Oxford was named as the man who shot at the Queen many years ago, and had subsequently been a patient in an asylum before he was discharged to Australia. He had recently been convicted of stealing a shirt and spent a week in jail. Upon his release, the prison governor had asked the police to keep an eye on him, 'in consequence of the old man's eccentric conduct'. To that end the police had arrested Oxford for vagrancy, and the article reported that he was up before the bench again. He was remanded for further medical examination. Haydon's update ended there.

This does not tally with other evidence about Oxford's time in Melbourne. In hindsight, it seems very likely that *The Age* had confused two would-be regicides. Their man John Oxford was more likely to have been John Francis, a man whose own crime echoed Oxford's in circumstances and mental state but whose gun was found to be loaded with more than powder. As a result,

Francis was found guilty of treason and dispatched to Australia rather than Bethlem. After spending several years a prisoner in Tasmania, he moved to Melbourne with only qualified success and constant money worries. Oxford by contrast had become a pillar of society. He was actually writing for *The Age* by 1880 under his new name of John Freeman, and his journalistic musings were later collated and published in book form as *Lights and Shadows of Melbourne Life*. Still a painter by trade he married, became a stepfather, was a churchwarden and also a senior officer of the West Melbourne Mutual Improvement Society. Though his doctors did not know it, Oxford had become a poster boy for asylum rehabilitation. His desire for recognition had been validated at last, even if the burden of his past would never quite disappear. Oxford told no one of his true identity, not even his wife, who mourned solely John Freeman when Oxford died in April 1900.

Oxford's death came only a few months before that of the woman who had been at the other end of his pistol in 1840. Victoria had survived not just Oxford and Francis, but several other assassination attempts during her reign. At the time of Oxford's trial, the government had feared that giving his case the oxygen of publicity would only fuel copycats, and so it came to pass. Mostly these came from subjects who, if not legally insane, were certainly considered by the general population to be mad. Their fates varied, and Broadmoor housed just one other: Roderick Maclean, who took his shot at the elderly monarch at Windsor Railway Station on 2 March 1882. A nomadic Scot, Maclean was also sentenced as a lunatic, but unlike Oxford he did not recover and remained at Broadmoor until his death in 1921.

Maclean's legacy was the change in sentence for those found to be criminal lunatics, from being 'not guilty by reason of insanity', to the more condemnatory 'guilty, but insane'. The motivation for the law change was always levelled at the Queen's alleged response to Maclean's not guilty verdict: 'Insane he may have been, but not guilty he most certainly was not, as I saw him fire the pistol myself'. This is a slight rewriting of history, as the Queen did not see Maclean shoot, though she did hear the report of his pistol. However, her displeasure at Maclean's innocence was real, and pressure was exerted on Prime Minister William Gladstone to change the law. It is unclear exactly what Victoria hoped to achieve by this, though Oxford was still in her mind. She suggested that if rather than be treated, he had been hanged all those years ago, it might have served to deter the potential killers who came after him: a rational suggestion, though not necessarily one to sway irrational minds. Forty years of being shot at had not mellowed Her Majesty.

3

Richard Dadd: Artist of Repute

Oxford is not the only well-known resident of Victorian Broadmoor. For many years, Richard Dadd was perhaps the most celebrated. Dadd's story is also timeless, run through as it is with that most recognisable trait of mental illness: delusions. Though Victorian psychiatry is a world away from how we consider the subject today, any nineteenth century alienist would immediately recognise the concept of delusions. Delusions were measurable, quantifiable and easily subject to peer review. They were usually coupled with a diagnosis of mania, and the joining of these two labels could be readily understood and witnessed by the layman to refer to someone who was 'obviously' mad.

Dadd was such a person, at least for most of his adult life. But not always. Before his illness took hold, he developed a reputation as an artist of some repute. The quality of his mythological paintings, in particular, was acknowledged during his lifetime, and he continued to paint remarkable works during his time in asylums. Many of these works survive, and quite apart from any sensational interest in Dadd's circumstances, it is accepted by many critics that Dadd possessed a rare talent.

His artistic endeavours had benefited from conducive surroundings. He was born into an intellectual family in Chatham, Kent, on 1 August 1817. Dadd's father, Robert, was a chemist and the first curator of the Chatham and Rochester Literary and Philosophical Institution's museum, and Dadd himself attended the King's

School at Rochester. Yet there were also clouds growing above the young man's head. Like Oxford, at a young age he lost a parent: in Dadd's case his mother Mary, who died when the boy was seven. Dadd was the fourth of seven children, four of whom would eventually die insane. His father remarried, but after he was widowed once more he moved the family to London, where he set up a business supplying art equipment.

Dadd was 17 when the family moved. Two years later, he was admitted to the Royal Academy Schools to train as an artist. Most of his work from this period is figurative, probably reflecting the life drawing that he studied. Various watercolours survive, which show family portraits and other people, who were both real and part of Dadd's everyday life.

At the same time, Dadd began to be influenced by literary and classical themes, and worked these up into canvases that he would submit for public exhibitions. These images were altogether different to the watercolour portraits, with their informal brush strokes and natural appearance. These fairy paintings, for which Dadd would become best known, were heavy in oil and intricately detailed, including characters with exaggerated expressions who populated fantastical backgrounds. They were very powerful works, and Dadd was noticed by the critics. In due course, he found a patron: Sir Thomas Phillips, a solicitor from South Wales, who had been knighted for his part in ending a Chartist riot, and had money to burn. Phillips decided that he wished to undertake the Grand Tour of classical sites across Europe, and he recruited Dadd to accompany him as his personal artist, and draw what they saw.

Because both men documented their journey it can be tracked in some detail. They set out on 16 July 1842, travelling first through Belgium, Germany and Switzerland before reaching Italy a month later. Here they began in earnest to soak up ancient culture, as they stopped in Venice and Bologna before taking a boat across the Adriatic to Corfu. From there, they wound their way across the Greek mainland, where another boat took them to Turkey, then on to Constantinople.

Dadd seemed to enjoy the tour, even though he had not enjoyed the breakneck speed at which they had arrived in the East, and he wrote various letters home detailing his wonderful experiences.

He was fascinated both by the scenery he encountered and the people he met, and an internal record of these compositions appears to have remained locked within him during his years of treatment. Decades later, scenes from his travels would still appear in the works he completed in Bethlem and Broadmoor.

Dadd's mind had been untethered and was running free across a new spiritual landscape. This process of liberation continued as the two tourists made their way through Syria and Palestine. Overwhelmed by vistas that seemed like 'pageants of a dream', the young man allowed himself to become a living sponge, saturated by the new world he was experiencing. He was struck, as well, by the comparative lack of etiquette and decorum compared to the constrained society that he knew at home. Challenges to his received wisdom were to be found round every corner, and it was all excellent stuff with which to fill an artist's head.

So far, so good. The tour itself was meeting expectations, although Phillips was still determined to continue apace. For him, this was an extended holiday before he returned to Britain, where his intention was to set up a legal practice in London. So within five months of setting off on a journey conducted solely over land and sea, Dadd and Phillips arrived in Egypt to embark on a Nile cruise. It was at this point that Dadd first began to exhibit signs of mental illness.

The evidence for this is within Dadd's letters home, where he wrote matter-of-factly about his increasingly weak grip on his old reality, coupled with his efforts to rationalise the source of his changing feelings. Overall, he was unconcerned. He recognised that the whole trip had placed him under great strain, even if it had been a marvellous experience. Yet while he and Phillips were on their boat, cruising upriver to Thebes then back down again, Dadd, for the first time since July, suddenly found that he had a lot of time on his hands. During this time, he allegedly suffered from sunstroke, affecting his mind, but perhaps it was rather that all the weight of experiences caught up with him and tipped his balance. A featherweight of paranoia and depression added itself to the contents of Dadd's pockets.

By February 1843, it was time to start the journey home. Dadd and Phillips left Cairo and sailed to Malta. It was another boat ride, and another deterioration in Dadd's state. He became bitterly depressed. Through Naples and then Rome, Dadd began to suspect that he was being watched. He was also suffering from delusions that there were anonymous parties conspiring to injure him. Coupled with this paranoia and fear were increasing signs of an obsession with religion. He experienced his first irrational impulse: to kill Pope Gregory XVI during a public appearance in Rome, an impulse he resisted as he felt the Pope was too well protected.

Dadd's head was becoming plagued by demons, which revealed themselves at inappropriate moments to frighten and confuse him. When the travellers reached Paris in May 1843 Dadd suffered a virtually complete breakdown, causing Phillips to send for a doctor to examine his travelling companion. Dadd panicked and fled home. Phillips wrote to the Dadd family to warn them that the man coming back to them was not one they would recognise. He was right. Dadd's demeanour was shocking in his description of his pursuit by spirits and his own desire to find the perpetrator of the sins committed against him.

Writing from Bethlem a few years later, Dadd summarised his position over that fateful summer: 'On my return from travel, I was roused to a consideration of subjects which I had previously never dreamed of ... and I had such ideas that, had I spoken of them openly, I must, if answered in the world's fashion, have been told I was unreasonable. I concealed, of course, these secret admonitions. I knew not whence they came, although I could not question their propriety, nor could I separate myself from what appeared to be my fate.'

His fate, it appeared, was twofold. Firstly, he was 'inclined to fall in with the views of the ancients ... coupled with the idea of a descent from the Egyptian god Osiris', and secondly, he was obliged to look for 'the Great Fiend', by which he meant the Devil. A delusion of being required to battle evil was common enough amongst Victorian lunatics, but in his kinship with Osiris Dadd was also presenting himself as the giver of eternal life and therefore hope to the dead. Not only was Osiris anciently linked with the sun, which came anew each day, but also the story of Osiris's betrayal, death and rebirth found echoes in future religions, and it became no less pivotal in their retelling. So it was that Dadd had now become touched by the resurrection. This gave him a position of great power and great responsibility. He began to exert a minute control over his own life, for instance insisting on only eating eggs and drinking beer, presumably to give him some degree of either purity or strength. He was also aware, more keenly than ever, that he was being watched. This was an inevitable consequence of his exalted position in the cosmos he felt, though it was also an inevitable consequence of the fact that his own friends and family had become increasingly worried about and wary of him.

At length, Robert Dadd was persuaded to consult Dr Alexander Sutherland of St Luke's Hospital, which was London's other hospital for the mad besides Bethlem. Sutherland came straight to the point: Dadd junior was dangerous and in need of immediate admission. Would Robert Dadd allow his son to be placed under Sutherland's care? If he was minded to do so, he did not act immediately, but instead responded to his son's consequent plea to 'unburthen his mind to him'. Richard suggested that they pay a visit to Cobham Park in Kent, close to Chatham and a scene of happier family memories for them both. His father agreed.

Unbeknown to Robert Dadd, it was becoming clearer and clearer to his son that evil was closer than he had ever realised. A picture was forming whereby members of his friends and family were in fact either 'The Great Fiend', or his representatives. For it was Dadd's friends and family who watched him most closely, and most imperilled his hunt for demons. This latest event merely reinforced this evidence. Now, his father was considering a plan to deny Dadd his very liberty, thus making it impossible for him to continue in his vital quest. It was time to take matters into his own hands.

Dadd was an intelligent man. Before meeting up with his father, he first obtained a passport and planned his getaway. Then they met on Monday, 28 August 1843, and found rooms for the night in separate cottages. They ate together, shared conversation and then before parting for the night walked out across Cobham Park, where Dadd attacked and killed his father, first trying to cut his throat with a razor, and finally stabbing him through the lung with a knife.

Dadd was aware that he had done something wrong, even if he was not exactly sure at this point who or what it was that he had killed. He followed his escape plan, and took a carriage down to Dover before hiring a boat to take him over to France. He later stated that he was on his way to kill the Emperor of Austria, but whatever the truth of that, he made his way to Paris, took another coach for Lyon, and within two days attacked a complete stranger who was his travelling companion. He was arrested by the French authorities and identified himself as a wanted man in England.

The law on insanity in France differed slightly to the law in England. In France, it was not necessary to bring the accused lunatic before a court to decide on whether he or she should plead; it was a decision solely for the doctors. So Dadd was examined in prison, explained that he was 'the son and envoy of God, sent to exterminate the men most possessed with the demon' and was eventually admitted to Clermont Asylum to the north of Paris.

Only after he had been received into custody did some explanation arise as to Dadd's motive for his acts. When he was arrested in France, the police had found on him a list of 'people who must die', with his father's name at the top. At around the same time, a search of his lodgings in England had uncovered various portraits of those close to him, all with a bloody slash painted across their throats. His attack on the French traveller had been caused by Dadd observing that two stars in the constellation of Ursa Major were moving closer together, and then taking that to be a sign that a further sacrifice was demanded by the ancient gods.

Notes from his stay at Clermont made clear Dadd's belief that his father was the Devil, and that he had been commanded to kill both Robert Dadd and 'many others'. The artist formerly known as Richard Dadd was now in fact a son of the sun, and spent 'entire days staring [at it] without blinking (so that the pupil remains slightly contracted)' in order to receive 'inspirations from above'. During these periods Dadd appeared to be in a form of religious ecstasy. This was balanced by the downside to his state of salvation, for Dadd was also compelled to suffer and then spit out the demons that sought to enter his body.

While Dadd resided as a guest of the French state, efforts were put in place by the Home Office to extradite him. These took the best part of a year, during which time Dadd's family sent food and art supplies to him. When Dadd was finally returned to England, in July 1844, by now with a long beard covering his face, he was certified by the Kent magistrates as insane and never required to enter a plea. This resulted in his immediate detention at Her Majesty's pleasure and so he was dispatched to the criminal lunatic ward at Bethlem. It was 22 August 1844, and Dadd would spend the rest of his life in asylum care.

Dadd arrived in a straitjacket, befitting his status as a dangerous lunatic, but in the few years since Oxford's trial John Conolly's ideas of non-restraint had become even more widely accepted and so the jacket was removed as soon as Dadd was in hospital care. Nevertheless, Dadd's world had now become very restricted. The accommodation for criminal lunatics at Bethlem was small: a four-storey annexe with galleries that doubled as dining and day rooms, with various rooms where the more violent clientèle found themselves allowed only to roam from their ten by eight foot box into a caged porch area. By day, the patients shared the multipurpose gallery or the small airing court, and by night they were locked into their own gloomy rooms. There was no delineation here between sufferers of different symptoms or those with different needs. Both the raving and the melancholy, the chronic and the recuperating, had to make do with the same cramped space.

Despite the potentially discouraging surroundings, almost immediately after he was confined to Bethlem Dadd began to paint again. It was a habit to be encouraged, as the pursuit of industry was a key plank of Victorian mental health care. There were few occupational facilities open to the Bethlem criminals and so any opportunity to gainfully employ a lunatic would have been gratefully taken. Dadd's virtuous habit was also one that would never leave him, and over the next 40 years he continued to develop the style and subjects that he had painted before the onset of his illness.

Dadd painted most of his more celebrated works while he was in Bethlem. Both 'The Fairy Feller's Master Stroke' and 'Oberon and Titania' date from his time there, although the former may have been completed in Broadmoor. These are usually considered to be the only fairy paintings that Dadd produced while in hospital, though the painstaking detail brushed onto each canvas meant that they took him several years to complete. The rest of Dadd's professional time was rather more occupied by his series of sketches 'to illustrate the Passions', a number of landscapes based upon his travels and also portraiture and literary artworks. Much of this work survives, and it has maintained a reputation for Dadd that sits apart from his madness. You do not have to be insane to appreciate the art of Richard Dadd, and nor does Dadd's insanity make his art any more or less brilliant.

Though his painting was a positive sign of well-being, Dadd found no cure for his illness at Bethlem under either of the two management phases that he experienced. The old, unaccountable Bethlem was finally given notice to improve by the Commissioners in Lunacy in 1852, after they had forcibly taken the private institution within the new, national regime of inspection and regulation. The idea was to drive up the standards of treatment. Before this time, record keeping was rather haphazard and medical intervention likewise, with doctors contracted as required by the hospital rather than permanently based on site. The commissioners concluded that it was impossible to know whether patient care was being maintained if there was no way of either guaranteeing or providing evidence for it.

The result was that Bethlem's first resident superintendent was appointed. Dr Charles Hood, fresh from medical school, was sent in to run the hospital in the modern, public asylum manner, as a refuge for its patients. He brought with him George Haydon, the equally young, well-travelled steward, who would be tasked with improving the surroundings and experience for the patient body.

Dadd was at least appreciated and possibly even encouraged by his new overlords. Hood had the energy of the reformer, and Haydon was a writer and an artist as well as a steward of lunatic asylums. Both men recognised Dadd's ability and collected work by him, with 'Oberon and Titania' dedicated to Hood and the 'Fairy Feller' to Haydon. They were Dadd's new patrons. Hood's appointment also coincided with the first notes being made at Bethlem on Dadd's condition. In March 1854 Hood summarised the case thus: 'For some years after his admission he was considered a violent and dangerous patient, for he would jump up and strike a violent blow without any aggravation and then beg pardon for the deed. This arose from some vague idea that filled his mind, and still does so to a certain extent, that certain spirits have the power of possessing a man's body and compelling him to adopt a particular course whether he will or no.' In Victorian terms, this sounded like a diagnosis of monomania, or delusions based around a specific subject.

Ten years had passed since Dadd had been admitted. Apart from work and routine, there was no strategic intervention that Victorian science could offer him, and unsurprisingly his mental state was unchanged. Once on the subject of the spirits, he would become 'excited in his manner of speaking' and 'unintelligible'. He also showed a determination to act in a manner that Hood described as 'perfectly a sensual being', which had been one of the key lessons brought home from his Grand Tour. Dadd continued to reject what he saw as the bonds of European society, and preferred to adopt a behavioural approach based on raw desire. Hood illustrated this by describing how Dadd would 'gorge himself with food until he actually vomits, and then return again to the meal'.

Dadd kept himself to himself at Bethlem, uninterested by the other patients and seemingly quiet and well-behaved. Despite this, Hood still reported that his patient was dangerous, and of course he was. Dadd's murderous urges had been confined rather than extinguished. If he had been discharged back into his previous society, his paranoia would probably have returned within weeks, if not days. In the asylum, he was unbothered by the conspiracy to deprive him of his god-like powers. This is worth noting. By no means all delusional patients absented their keepers from responsibility for their condition, but Dadd appears to have done so.

Hood and Haydon succeeded in improving things a little for their criminal lunatics, and indeed Hood was even able to find space to separate the guilty, convict patients from the innocent but insane in 1857. Bethlem was moving on, and its new ways would have prepared Dadd for his move to the wide expanses of Broadmoor, where patients of different symptoms and behaviour were more likely to be housed apart than together; where there were day rooms, gardens and vistas aplenty; and where the whole operation was managed with a closer attention to detail. In theory, the set up was much more in harmony with Dadd's needs.

Dadd was one of the last batch of Bethlem patients to make the journey down to Crowthorne. He made the great trek to the Berkshire countryside on 23 July 1864, a few days short of his forty-seventh birthday and with five other men for company. A soldier and four labourers, these were all pleasure men like him who had watched as their previous accommodation gradually became vacant. It must have been a curious summer, for every few days another handful of faces disappeared from the gallery and the criminal wing was slowly wound down. At the end of the day that Dadd departed London, the state asylum at Bethlem lay empty.

In his new asylum, Dadd was soon examined and interviewed. He was still convinced of his delusions, believing himself to be 'a marked man under the influence of an evil spirit'. His interviewer, probably William Orange, recorded that Dadd: 'Makes laboured attempts at justification of the two criminal assaults saying it was in "justification of the Deity".' There was no change in Dadd's belief system from 20 years ago, and nor would there ever be.

Dadd settled in to his new accommodation quickly and began painting again. By November 1864 he was engaged in a watercolour fairy scene, most likely a copy of the 'Fairy Feller'. Dadd followed up the watercolour with a long poem based on the original work, which may well have been sent to Haydon and was later purchased by the Bethlem archives. Then Dadd moved back to his mystical travelling scenes.

His drive and motivation seems to have been a very personal thing. Although he was not the only artist in Victorian Broadmoor, he was easily the most talented and had no proper competition. The handful of other professionals during Dadd's stay had all failed to match his output while in care, or to make a successful career of their calling. Only one, a London sculptor called Richard Wheeler, appears to have carried on drawing systematically at Broadmoor. It is also a myth to suppose that Dadd worked surrounded by creative types: Wheeler was in a different block and the other painters, actors and writers in the patient group were spread around the male side. Dadd was probably in blissful ignorance of most kindred passengers on the site, and if he engaged at all with comrades at the easel then his choice was probably restricted to the members of a band of willing amateurs. The most satisfactory conclusion is that Dadd thought and drew alone.

Perhaps he thrived because of his surroundings rather than in spite of them.

His physical health was his principal burden. Dadd suffered from gout from time to time, though his attacks were short-lived and he was usually able to keep up an intake of wine and spirits during these periods. But during 1868 to 1870 he suffered a prolonged bout of illness. In August 1868 he was removed to the infirmary in Block 3, with a severe fever and a depressed view of his own chances of survival believing that 'it is quite time'. He stayed there for a little over a month, complaining that an 'animal inside him' was devouring all the food he took, before he was able to be moved back to his room to recuperate. It was obviously a serious virus, as by 1870 he was still being given additional food and was recorded as having lost three stone over the past two years. However, he had recovered sufficiently by 1872 to begin to paint decorations for and around the stage in Broadmoor's central hall, which he continued for several years. There were other gifts too for the hospital, such as murals on the walls; some decorative figures on glass panels; a handful of watercolour caricatures; and the 'Portrait of a Broadmoor Officer'. The latter, dating from 1875, was long supposed to be a likeness of William Orange, though it may well be of Dadd's 29-year-old doctor and Orange's deputy at the time, David McKay Cassidy. It was Cassidy who was writing up Dadd's case notes in 1875, and though he left Broadmoor later that year, Cassidy sent Dadd five pounds in February 1878, which may well have been to settle a debt for work done. Even if Orange was not the subject of the portrait, he was not to be left out and he received his own present: a mural painted along one wall in the medical superintendent's house, now lost, like most of Dadd's hall decorations.

Dadd's continuing output hints at a man who was presumably content. For Dadd was a tranquil patient, whose madness only became apparent during conversations on the usual topics. His notes regularly state his seeming contentment with his position, as well as the stubborn continuation of his delusions. One conversation with Dadd, written up by Orange shortly after Dadd arrived was on the subject of chess and how some people possessed a spirit that allowed them to play 'without the board'. Dadd further mused that chess pieces could be unfriendly towards some players due to the 'antiquity of the game'. Similarly, when he was taken ill with fever Dadd concluded this was due to the heat of the sun, and that as a mad person he had no 'spirit to intercede' for him against its rays. As a result, he was bound to suffer the sun god's punishment.

Only one note was made at Broadmoor relating to the direct cause of Dadd's admission. In 1877 David Nicolson recorded a detailed conversation about Robert Dadd's murder, which now included the mythology that Richard had used to interpret the scene. Dadd stated that he was not convinced that the man he killed had been his father, presumably clinging to the belief that he had instead attacked the Devil. Rather, Dadd had been convinced at the time of the killing that the 'gods and spirits above' required him to make a sacrifice. 'Dadd', wrote Nicolson, '(posing himself with upstretched arm), thus apostrophised the starry bodies "Go," said he "and tell the great god Osiris that I have done the deed which is to set him free".' It was a heroic story and would have been a worthy subject for a Dadd canvas.

Despite his continuing delusions, Dadd was evidently no trouble to the medical authorities. He remained insane, but in other respects simply became another old man, occasionally wandering about the grounds to watch the other patients playing cricket. His disappearance underneath the asylum radar is evidenced by the fact that no entries were made on his case for seven years, from 1878 until 1885, at which point he was removed to the infirmary in Block 3 with what proved to be his final illness. It was back to where Dadd had spent his first years in Broadmoor, mingling with the patients who were not overtly dangerous but could also not be entirely trusted. He had obviously been one of Block 3's better behaved patients, as he was not required to suffer a dormitory, but had his own room. At some point, he was almost certainly moved into Block 2, the privilege block where only the most independent patients were placed, as he appeared there in a journalist's report made in the 1880s. Perhaps he was moved at the same point as he stopped being observed, left quietly to manage his own affairs and entertain himself.

For what does survive of this part of Dadd's life are his personal accounts, which show that he was not simply bricked up and forgotten. He received money from the occasional paying customer, as well as wages for his hospital work, and in the patients' account books Dadd's careful, slow signature records both those receipts and the expenditure on millboard, paper, and brushes that he purchased for his work. Nor were these the only treats that Dadd purchased for himself: there were books, particularly classical and religious texts; sweets such as peppermints and barley sugars; as well as other foods with strong flavours, like herrings and gingerbread, which Dadd may well have bought to augment the bland asylum food. These purchases show someone who enjoyed life enough to want to take an active part in what it had to offer, even if he was limited in what that offer was.

When the first note was made on Dadd's case for seven years, it was to say that he had complained of feeling unwell. It was June 1885 and he had acquired tuberculosis, probably from one of the other patients. He was removed to the infirmary and spent six months there and in the Block 4 sick ward until his death on the evening of 8 January 1886, aged 68. The end had been quick, with Dadd still getting up and about until a week before he died. When he was gone, the Broadmoor clerk wrote to his sister-in-law as next of kin, as only she had remained in occasional touch with the doctors if not with Dadd himself. Such situations were common in Broadmoor. Like a significant proportion of asylum patients, Dadd had outlived most of his immediate family, and there were no close relatives left to mourn his passing. His body was not reclaimed, and he was buried in the asylum cemetery. Organising what possessions remained in his estate proved a harder task. Letters in Dadd's Broadmoor file indicate that 11 years after his death, these possessions still had not been dispersed, nor had the 15 pounds left credited to Dadd's account. The file concludes by noting that various solicitors' letters had been taken from it by the Broadmoor steward, sadly never to be returned.

Dadd's true surviving legacy was his work, though this also took a little time to become apparent. For while Dadd's reputation was recognised during his lifetime, due to his situation he was not particularly celebrated and only rarely exhibited. He was a slight embarrassment to the world of art, which was unsure what to say about him. His passing was not noted when he died, and the first major exhibition of his work was only curated in 1974, at The Tate in London. Forty years later and Dadd has become an established

Victorian name. The Tate holds various paintings, among them 'The Fairy Feller's Master Stroke', and a substantial collection of his work is held at the Bethlem Royal Hospital Museum, including the paintings that remained at Broadmoor after Dadd's death. A lost work, 'The Artists' Halt in the Desert', was discovered in 1987, during filming for the BBC's *Antiques Roadshow*, and is now in The British Museum, and there are still plenty of other known works which are missing and yet to be rediscovered. Interest in Dadd's work has only deepened with time, and there seems little chance that this particular artist will ever be forgotten.

4

William Chester Minor: Man of Words and Letters

For many years, Richard Dadd was the best-known Victorian Broadmoorite to achieve success despite his position. Oxford's good works in Australia had not yet been noticed, and no other patient had been marked as contributing to Victorian society from within the asylum walls. That changed with Simon Winchester's best-selling book *The Surgeon of Crowthorne*, which shone a very bright light on to Dr William Chester Minor, an American medic, murderer and contributor to the first Oxford English Dictionary. Minor demonstrated a different strain of creativity to Dadd, but one no less incredible in its accomplishment.

Minor had an unconventional upbringing. Born in Ceylon on 22 June 1834, he was the son of a couple of Christian missionaries who had been called to the Jaffna Peninsula from a rather comfortable background in the United States. Eastman and Lucy Minor joined the various American immigrants in the far north of the island, where they were contained by the ruling British from venturing further south. As well as proselytising to the resident Tamil population, the missionaries built schools and hospitals and also focused on language: part of their work was to translate texts into Tamil and then print them, and it was with this that Eastman Minor had arrived to help.

Minor never knew his mother, for Lucy died from tuberculosis when the boy was two. Tragically, she became the first person to be buried in the American Mission's new cemetery at Uduvil, just to the north of Jaffna city. Faced with the prospect of being sole carer for William and his newborn sister, Eastman Minor took off to Singapore, where he found a new partner. William travelled with him. On their return, Eastman remarried and went on to have a further eight children. Minor lived with his new family until he reached the age of 14, being schooled by the mission and surrounded by books. Then, his father decided that the boy should return home for his education and he was packed off to live with his aunt and uncle in New Haven, Connecticut.

New Haven was rather different to the rural island that Minor had left. It was an urban centre of manufacturing, home to tens of thousands of people. Nevertheless, he was now safe in the bosom of his extended, middle-class family, where he remained until his father and stepmother finally returned from Ceylon in 1852.

Minor's teenage years are his least well documented, though it seems reasonable to assume that they were formative, and not necessarily in a positive way. Because, for all his love of words, Minor's real obsession was with sex. At the time it was probably unremarkable. He was a young man, after all, and he would have been far odder if he had not been interested in the subject. Also, he would have had little opportunity to practise apart from by himself, though he may well have had the first inkling that for him desire was always to be accompanied by paralysing guilt.

In his early twenties, Minor was accepted at the local university, Yale, where he studied medicine. He worked hard, specialised in anatomy, and graduated in 1863, which was a time of great domestic upheaval in the US. The Civil War was raging. Minor felt his own call, and walked straight into it. In June, he joined the Union Army as a surgeon and less than a year later found himself experiencing his first active service on the battlefield. In the context of the Civil War, Minor's trauma was not too great: he spent a short time at the Battle of the Wilderness – a fierce and bloody engagement – but was then moved back from the front line and spent the rest of the war tending to the wounded who had survived the field hospitals and been transported nearer home for treatment.

Minor enjoyed his service enough to continue it. At the end of the Civil War, he remained in the army and indeed rose through the ranks to become a captain. Then in 1866 he moved to a hospital at Governors Island, New York, and it is here that the first signs of illness were detected. Several years later, when Minor was on trial, his half-brother George reported that Minor told him he had been forced to brand a deserter, and that his victim felt 'he had done it with unnecessary severity'. As a result, Minor said that he had become a 'marked man'. There was also an episode of sunstroke, which together with the death of his father was blamed for his change of character. But these arguments for the defence were typical crises presented on the Victorian lunatic's behalf, and they were also perfectly polite defences to be articulated in a public hearing.

What was not put forward at his trial was Minor's very own elephant in the room: sex. He began daily to frequent brothels in New York, where he acquired venereal infections. Even within the bounds of what might be considered normal for a soldier, or tacitly encouraged, there was obviously something about Minor's behaviour that was troubling. With the benefit of hindsight, it is likely that he was engaging in either homosexual or bisexual acts as well as more traditional forms of prostitution, and he was not able to accept his needs. A host of fears made him their guest, in addition to very real diseases. Not only was he overcome by lust, but his preferred forms of satisfaction were forbidden by scripture. In these circumstances it was not surprising if he was being divinely punished through illness. However, there was a more disturbing consequence of Minor's nightly assignations. It seemed very likely to Minor that he was being watched, and it did not take a great leap of irrational thought to suppose that the people who were following his carnal crimes might also be responsible for his suffering. Convinced that there were dark forces raised against him, Minor began to carry his gun around.

He was moved to Florida, where the sunstroke incident befell him, but matters did not improve. Minor challenged a colleague to a duel. By now, he was seeing persecution around every corner. In September 1868, he was diagnosed with delusional monomania and shortly afterwards was sent to the Government Hospital for the Insane in Washington DC, now known as St Elizabeth's Hospital, where he stayed until he was formally retired from the army in April 1871.

William Chester Minor: Man of Words and Letters

In receipt of a pension, Minor returned home to New Haven and to George, a reunion lasting all of three months. Every night, Minor heard noises in the house, and every night he saw people in his room. These intruders were only after two things: first to drug him, and then to use his body in the most depraved ways imaginable. Each morning at the breakfast table Minor would dissect the vile happenings of the night before.

George suggested that the solution to Minor's situation might be to go to Europe. Minor had always wanted to travel, and like Dadd to take the Grand Tour. With his pension and a family allowance, money was no obstacle to Minor following one of his dreams. So it was with some relief in Connecticut, though not a little trepidation, that William Chester Minor set off from Boston in the autumn of 1871.

Minor disembarked in London and never made it any further. He took up residence at Vidler's Hotel in Holborn, before moving to Lambeth after Christmas, almost certainly so that he could have easier access to the capital's sex trade. The subsequent series of events was tragically inevitable. First of all, Minor approached Scotland Yard, reporting that he was being followed and otherwise persecuted by various nameless Irishmen. The warning was ignored. Minor then made several visits to reaffirm his problem. By now he was convinced that his nightly visitors, who were all male at this point, were intent on killing him with poison. Minor wrote letters to the police on the subject, though neglecting to tell them that he had imported his pistol within his luggage. The police considered him to be insane but otherwise harmless.

They were wrong. One night in February 1872 Minor woke, and saw an imaginary figure at the end of the bed. Finding himself to be free from the stupor of drugs, Minor decided to confront his abuser. When it did not answer him, but ran, he pursued the phantom spirit into the street, where Minor chanced upon a real man called George Merritt who was walking to work at a brewery near Waterloo. Merritt was married and had six children, with another on the way, and that night he was simply in the wrong place at the wrong time. Minor chased him, pursued him as he ran, and then caught and shot at him twice, once in the chest and again in the neck.

The scene of crime was very central, between Waterloo and Hungerford bridges, and Minor was apprehended on the spot. Minor said it was a case of self-defence, that he had thought Merritt was a person who had forced entry to his room. He realised now that it was also a case of mistaken identity, and that Merritt was not the man he thought he had seen. While the mistake was fleeting, its consequences were permanent. Merritt was dead.

Minor was committed for trial, and this was held at the Surrey Assizes in Kingston upon Thames in April 1872. As well as the mention of sunstroke and branding, there was adequate evidence for the true nature of Minor's enduring delusions. A warder at the jail where Minor was on remand was also an employee at Bethlem, and he testified that every morning Minor would wake up and level the accusation that his guards had allowed men into his room at night. His abusers were cunning fellows, and they hid in the voids of the room, under the bed or in the walls or rafters. The fiends in this retelling were always male, but both men and women, boys and girls featured in Minor's later descriptions of the sexual terrors that his abusers forced upon him nightly. This was the subject of his monomania, and had been since his first diagnosis by the US Army. A hundred years later, Minor would have been described as a paraphrenic, or paranoid schizophrenic. There was the mention also that it was all punishment for an unspecified act that Minor had been forced to endure while in the Union Army; perhaps this was when Minor had felt violated for the first time.

Whatever Minor's confused reasoning for his actions, the jury believed that he was not guilty by reason of insanity. He duly received the sentence of detention at Her Majesty's pleasure, and was sent straight to Broadmoor. Minor arrived from the Surrey County Gaol on 17 April 1872. Unusually for a Broadmoor patient, he travelled with another patient being transferred from the same prison, a gentleman called Edmund Dainty, who had killed a man in the Surrey Asylum and been tried at the same assizes. Described on admission as 'a thin, pale and sharp-featured man with light coloured sandy hair; deep-set eyes and prominent cheek bones', Minor dutifully recounted his persistent nocturnal experiences, as well as giving an account of his current bodily health (gonorrhoea and possible signs of tuberculosis, though none were found). Like Dadd, his delusions appeared to be self-contained and manageable. He was obviously thought to be a low risk and was placed in Block 2, where privileges and independence were greatest.

There was another factor at play in Minor's speedy move to the privilege block. He was an American citizen. The Consulate in London had tried to help him at his trial, and almost as soon as he arrived in the asylum, they wrote to William Orange for permission to send various things to Minor: both his own possessions and 'some comforts, such as Dunn's Coffee, French Plums etc'. The Consulate also sent on Minor's retrieved possessions shortly after, including his clothes, drawing equipment, his tobacco and his diary. They kept hold of his surgical instruments, which had also been found in his rooms.

As a patient in Block 2, Minor enjoyed a reasonable degree of freedom within the hospital routine. He had a generous, regular income from his family which allowed him, on a much larger scale than Dadd, to ask the hospital to purchase things for him. Minor consumed quantities of groceries daily – meat, poultry, fish, cakes and biscuits, coffee. He had his own wardrobe and a copious supply of art materials, allowing him to continue his proficiency at landscape painting. He played the flute, and at least one receipt survives for a tailor-made instrument he had supplied by Rudall Carte of London. He also regularly purchased newspapers and a number of engineering journals – the latter quite possibly for advice about concrete building construction, which he thought might prevent his nightly suffering.

Then there were his books. Like Prospero, Minor had at least been exiled with his personal library. It seems very likely that his family shipped his books to him, though he also purchased new ones. The library grew to such an extent that at some point after 1876, when Orange succeeded in having most of the convict patients transferred out, Minor was allowed a separate day room in which to store his books. This was some luxury, and Minor continued to be accorded it long after the asylum began to refill with patients.

The location of Minor's rooms is unfortunately lost in the mists of time, though within the hospital itself the received wisdom is that Minor had his suite on the top, second floor of Block 2, from which he would have had a fine view of the Broadmoor grounds. The rooms were certainly separate from each other, though probably close together, as the staff would not have wanted Minor to be a resident of multiple wards. For exceptionally, there is a suggestion that Minor may have had his own key to the day room. A note in his file from 1887 suggests that Minor could not get in one morning, as the lock was faulty (which no doubt provided him with further evidence of the shadows who raged against him), and he had to wait outside until the attendants had removed an obstruction from it.

There is comparatively little in the way of such revelatory notes in Minor's Broadmoor file, as his day-to-day privileges were simply that. Much of the anecdotal evidence for them comes from a 1958 letter written by Dr Patrick McGrath, then the superintendent. McGrath reported on a conversation with the daughter of David Nicolson, who had known Minor for 20 years. She confirmed most of the details above, as well as reporting that Minor had a private stock of wines and spirits, played the flute about the wards, and would from time to time dine with her family in the superintendent's home. It was an existence as comfortable as that of any Broadmoor patient, and one of the few relevant gleanings from the official paperwork confirms the picture of Minor as Broadmoor's college don. In 1901 there is a note about his employment of another patient as his servant. Such an arrangement depended on a suitable employee being available, of course, and the nature of admission and discharge meant that Minor would occasionally have to change his domestic staff. Presumably the attendants head-hunted on his behalf and then one lucky candidate from lower down the social orders found himself a ready wage with which to buy his own indulgences.

With cash to spend and plenty of time to kill, Minor began to amass books and read voraciously. It was for this obsession that he would come to be remembered in a positive light. In 1879, Sir James Murray embarked on his own obsession of creating the first Oxford English Dictionary, and placed an 'appeal to English speakers and the English reading public' for help. Murray needed examples of words and word use. Minor must have come across this appeal in one of his newspapers and felt a calling of his own.

He wrote to offer his services, and soon after began a regular series of submissions to the dictionary staff, contributing what became thousands of examples of word use from his book collection to assist their Herculean labours.

Minor was a very important contributor to the dictionary and much appreciated by Murray. Through his work, the two men met. Indeed, an apocryphal account of their first meeting has been around for some time, invented by a journalist called Hayden Church, who reported that Murray had been determined to visit Crowthorne after Minor had failed to turn up to a celebratory dinner in Oxford. Shocked to find himself arriving at a postal address shared by England's best-known asylum, Murray was received by Dr Nicolson, then the medical superintendent, whereupon Murray made the obvious conclusion; if he was facing a doctor, then that doctor must be Minor. Murray thanked Nicolson for his contribution to the dictionary. Nicolson of course corrected Murray and assured him that it was not he that should be thanked, whereupon Murray was walked from the central block to Block 2, through the corridors of what presumably were howling lunatics (or at least, painting, reading and writing lunatics), up the stairs and into Minor's day room. Murray's reaction was to gasp through his generous beard in amazement.

The truth is rather less dramatic. Certainly, Murray knew who and what he was visiting long before he made the journey down from his home in London. Broadmoor was hardly a secret, and even if Murray inhabited a closeted scholarly world, a quick glance by Murray's staff in any county directory would have been enough to confirm that Minor was not on the staff at Broadmoor. What seems more plausible is that Murray was aware of his contributor's situation and had considered him to be out of bounds until he realised that someone else had visited him in Crowthorne. Simon Winchester quotes a letter from Murray suggesting this possibility, as within it Murray writes that he remained unaware of Minor's past until the late 1880s, when an American librarian told him all. This is perhaps a half-remembering that paints its subject in a better light.

The first letter from Murray in Minor's file is dated 3 January 1891, and confirms the time of their first meeting. It hints at an earlier exchange between Murray and Nicolson, and in it Murray confirmed that he wished to make arrangements to visit Minor for the first time. Nicolson had evidently invited both men to lunch at his house.

There is no record of this meeting in the Broadmoor archive. Murray's letter mentioned above suggests that both before and after their lunch the two men spent time together alone in Minor's day room, where presumably the latter's library was examined in some detail. Murray would have found Minor to be an interesting companion, though if the conversation had turned to Minor's health it seems very unlikely that the monomania would not have been apparent.

The two men formed some sort of connection, even if the extent of Minor and Murray's relationship afterwards remains open to conjecture. They certainly corresponded, but evidence from Minor's file suggests that they met only sporadically. When Murray wrote to Dr Brayn on 21 August 1901, he reflected that he had not seen Minor since just before Nicolson retired. That places their previous meeting towards the end of 1895, and implies that at the time of writing, Murray had not visited Minor for six years. It was probably not the key relationship in either man's life that it has been portrayed as.

While Minor's enthusiasm for the written word was a source of great value to him, his books would also come to play a part in the regular refinement and updating of his delusions. From 1884, the agents of his degradation were defacing them at night, so that he would find them the next day presumably shot through with lewdness and immorality. This new twist followed an advance from chloroform being used at night, rendering him helpless to abuse and humiliation, to the application of electricity. Minor was not alone amongst the delusional lunatics to make use of technological advances. Poison could just as easily be administered through power as through potions, and discoveries in the world of telecommunications afforded many opportunities for the irrational mind to become subject to their influence.

Minor's books were the most sacred thing to him after his body, and now both were at risk. He was powerless to prevent harm and it is to his credit that he somehow managed to control his own fear and continuing working. For Minor must have found the approach of night a very frightening thing, as it brought with it the certainty of pain and guilt. His case notes provide some insight into his bedtime routine: he would barricade his room every night by placing furniture across the door. That would never work, of course. Only very occasionally would the attendants report that his nights had not been restless; usually, the morning brought fresh reports of his sordid trials. He expended much effort on trying to remedy the situation through practical means, such as the barricade, by asking the superintendent to keep a close watch on the attendants and so on. He was also always open to offering other solutions to try and retain some power over his torments. For example, the following letter was sent to Orange on 6 October 1884:

'Dear Sir

Let me mention one fact that falls in with my hypothesis. So many fires have occurred in the US originating quite inexplicably in the interspace of ceiling and floor; that I learn now Insurance Companies refuse to insure large buildings – mills, factories etc – which have the usual hollow spacing under the floor. They insist upon solid floors. All this has come to notice within ten years; but no one suggests any explanation.

Very sincerely yours,

WC Minor'

Orange had no budget to rebuild Block 2, even if he had wished to undertake the futile act. Minor was obviously cared for, though. Both Orange and Nicolson would bring their own guests to see him, quite apart from the interest in him taken by his family and friends. In addition to his regular allowance of around £100 a year he received regular correspondence from his step-family, as well as letters from friends of the family and other friends that he seems to have made after his sentencing. His file also contains the occasional notes of visits from London acquaintances who had travelled down for the day, as well as evidence that travellers from the United States came to see him. The latter included his old commanding officer in the army.

Sir James Murray wrote about another visitor: Eliza Merritt, the widow of George. Murray reported Nicolson as saying that Minor sent money to Mrs Merritt, and that she occasionally visited him. It is an intriguing proposition, and though Simon Winchester alludes to notes that Orange made upon Minor and Eliza's first meeting, there is no evidence to suggest either payments from Minor's account or visits in the Broadmoor archive. Indeed, there might be reason to conclude that there was motive for neither: a public subscription after George Merritt's murder had raised over £200 for the family, and Mrs Merritt herself was given a pension by the brewery where her husband worked. She did not remarry, and as a single parent to seven children – the youngest of whom was born shortly after her husband's death – it would probably have been some years before she would have had the time to give priority to a visit to her husband's killer. Perhaps if money changed hands then it was from the Minor family's accounts; perhaps if Minor and Eliza ever met then this was a solitary happening.

The portrait of Minor as a popular, entertaining man has to be balanced against his persistently challenging behaviour. Mostly this had its origins in the usual problems, and so it was that the attendants would be regularly accused of either molesting Minor, or of allowing him to be molested. Sometimes it was plain stubbornness, such as Minor's refusal to come inside during a snowstorm in January 1897: 'I am allowed to go out and can choose my own weather'.

But Minor's condition was also deteriorating. This could often only be realised at intervals, as reading his notes gives the impression that he tried to internalise his feelings until the pressure was too great, and then he would suddenly explode, making an accusatory outburst to the attendants or the superintendent. The most catastrophic example of this was when he eventually took matters into his own hands. On the morning of 3 December 1902 he tied a tourniquet around the base of his penis and sliced off the offending organ. He was 68 years old, and had never been able to come to terms with his own sexual urges. Asked why he had done it, he replied, "In the interests of morality". Minor's reasoning was that if he could no longer have sex, then he would no longer be taken out of the asylum at night and forced to fornicate with between 50 and 100 women "from Reading to Land's End." He spent time in the infirmary while he recovered, but was discharged after four months back to Block 2. Sadly of course, his retaliatory act against himself did not defeat his delusions, which remained as prevalent as before. In his last letter to Dr Brayn, shortly before his discharge, Minor was complaining still of 'these nightly sensual uses of my body that I experience and struggle against'.

As suggested earlier, the nature of these 'sensual uses' may provide some help in understanding Minor and his mental illness. Winchester's book suggests various hypotheses about Minor's own sexual motivations, from dusky eastern maidens with pert breasts to disease and prostitution in New York's metropolis, and to some form of sexual guilt about his feelings for Eliza Merritt. However, Minor's early delusions at Broadmoor all seem to relate to his body being used by men, and it is only in the later years that women play the more significant part. To the modern reader, Minor may be repressing homosexual, or even paedophiliac tendencies as much as heterosexual ones. Plenty of things may have happened to Minor before he came to the attention of the authorities, though we may never know exactly what Minor's own sexual experiences were, and how his obsessions became part of his developing illness. What is beyond doubt is that Minor was able to concoct outrageous tales of depravity, experienced with a multitude of other bodies, of both sexes and all ages, and that his mutilation of his own body was a direct result of his discomfort with that fact.

Still riddled with fear and hampered by his lifelong burdens, Minor had also become a very old and frail man, which brought additional problems. His family had recognised this, and after his stepbrother Alfred assumed control of Minor's affairs in 1897, more efforts were put into trying to bring the old man home. They were helped in part by an increasing catalogue of unfortunate incidents: there was the peotomy; a bath where Minor neglected to check the water temperature and severely scalded himself; and then a serious bout of influenza. Though initially unreceptive to the idea of discharge, by 1903, Richard Brayn was suggesting to Minor's stepbrother that a proposal to remove Minor to America might be received favourably, providing suitable care could be found for him.

It took seven years before matters reached a resolution, though it is unclear why: perhaps the family were having trouble finding a US hospital that they liked. In the meantime Minor became more and more decrepit. In 1909 and 1910, Brayn felt compelled from time to time to remove Minor to the infirmary, not thinking it safe to leave Minor alone in his room day after day, as he was no longer capable of looking after himself. Laid up, and deprived of his books and his art materials, Minor was increasingly miserable, as well as increasingly harmless. The tipping point for everyone came when Minor managed to complete a painting for the Princess of Wales but was not allowed to send it to her. He complained to what had now become the American Embassy. Finally, in April 1910 a conditional discharge was granted for his release. Both Sir James and Lady Murray visited him one last time before he was escorted to the Tilbury Docks on 15 April (via Bracknell, Waterloo and St Pancras), where he was put on board a steamer and handed over to the care of Alfred for the journey back across the Atlantic.

After 38 years in Broadmoor, Minor found himself arriving back in America only to be immediately returned to the Government Hospital for the Insane in Washington. In the end, no other accommodation had been forthcoming. So it was that he swapped one similar regime for another: a private room, certain privileges, and still the nightly torments. Though the Broadmoor authorities had thought he was nearing the end of his life, he managed to keep going for a further decade, reading, writing, and making the occasional outburst. He remained in Washington until November 1919, when he was compassionately discharged to be nearer his family, at the Retreat for the Elderly Insane in Hartford, Connecticut. He died there on 26 March 1920.

Inevitably for Minor there has to be a postscript, because unlike Dadd, whose work was at least acknowledged during his lifetime, Minor's place in history has only been secured after his death. Hayden Church, the author of the imagined Minor/Murray first meeting, published that first romantic piece about Minor in 1915 and another in 1944. He intended to write a book about Minor – there is a relevant letter in Minor's file stating this intention – but eventually did not. Then in the 1980s the Oxford University Press began to show a greater interest in its own history and of Minor's place within it, and a more scholarly article about the American army surgeon in Crowthorne was published. This in turn attracted Simon Winchester to write a full biography which spread the story around the world. Once it had happened, it seemed like an obvious conclusion to the tale: Minor's story is ultimately one of triumph in adversity, with a dose of sex and a grisly murder, and that combination always makes for a good read.

To a certain extent Minor has become a man of myth and legend, as obscure as any of the archaic words that he revisited for Sir James Murray's masterpiece. This seems a shame, because there is a real person tucked away inside the legend, and undoubtedly more to discover in this case about both him and Victorian society. There is also the story of the Merritt family, who grew up without their father through the very rare harming of a stranger by a foreigner with mental illness: a fact that makes Minor an unlikely hero, and is itself worthy of reflection. For though Minor may have been the richest immigrant in Victorian Broadmoor, he was not alone.

5

Broadmoor's International Brigade

While Minor is the best known example of a Victorian lunatic who came from overseas, a small number of other patients at Broadmoor also fitted this description. These patients were represented within the walls of Victorian Broadmoor in the same slim proportion as in the outside world. Of course, by far the greater number of patients had been born within the Home Nations: England, Wales, Scotland, Ireland or even the Channel Islands. It was far more unusual to find a naturalised Briton from more exotic climes, or a foreigner who had barely set foot in the country before feeling the long arm of the law. Yet these patients did exist.

For Broadmoor reflected the wide reach of Victorian England in attracting trade and immigrants from across the globe. This economic powerhouse sucked in resources to the docks of London and other ports, where ships would come from far away to load or unload. There were no restrictions either as to who might wish to make England their home. With no laws on immigration, anyone was welcome to try their luck in expanding Albion. It was almost inevitable that the population of Broadmoor did not belong to one homogenous culture, and that a handful of patients had ended up in asylum care from rather unexpected places.

The question of why these patients found a home in the first criminal lunatic asylum for England and Wales is one of legal jurisdiction. Broadmoor's national status meant that it would take admissions from the judicial system in both countries. Some

Broadmoor's International Brigade

foreign nationals, like Minor, were caught up in this process, finding themselves far from home at their time of crisis. Others discovered that the court system did not distinguish between ethnic backgrounds and then, as now, a minority of the indigenous lunatics of England and Wales could trace their roots back to places far away from the British Isles. Their stories are all unique, but some examples give a broader picture of their experiences.

As might be expected of a group who had travelled across land and sea to make their fortune, virtually all of the international brigade were male. They began arriving in Crowthorne as soon as Broadmoor opened, and were part of the same transfers that brought Oxford and Dadd to the asylum. These early days saw comparatively huge numbers of admissions for the staff to process, as roughly three times a week another small batch of patients and their attendants arrived at Wokingham Station on the train from Bethlem. The initial members of Broadmoor's international brigade were among them. Auguste Widmer arrived first on 2 March, followed three days later by John Flinn and Miguel Yzquierdo, and at the end of the month, William Stolzer. Each one of these gentlemen's stories provides a reference point for those who came after them.

The first of these names to be entered into the admissions register, Widmer had arrived at Bethlem in January 1861, at the age of 35. He had been found insane at the Middlesex Sessions on a charge of housebreaking in Charlotte Street, Westminster, and detained indefinitely at Her Majesty's pleasure. Widmer immediately, if inadvertently, demonstrated to the Bethlem staff an added complication of the overseas patient. No one could communicate with him, as Widmer spoke French and no English, and for them the position was reversed. Although it might be thought undesirable for a sick man to have no way of making himself understood, the staff at Bethlem did not attempt to resolve the situation. Widmer was isolated on the criminal lunatic ward in Southwark with little company, and it was only when he arrived at Broadmoor a few years later that the more cosmopolitan staff employed in Berkshire were able to converse with him. As it transpired, this had only a limited benefit. He told them that he was a cabinet maker from Zurich, in Switzerland, and after that brief flurry of biography he was not inclined to offer much further information. In truth, it now seemed unlikely that the years of oral isolation at Bethlem had been a burden to him, and it was his preference to remain a quiet and solitary patient. Widmer never learnt to speak any English and eventually refused to respond to the staff in French either. He was prone to outbursts of violence when he felt that he was being persecuted, and he ended up permanently in one of the refractory blocks, often in seclusion. He also took to running away from the medical staff if they approached him, and as a result even when he was not secluded, he spent most of his time at Broadmoor on his own.

There was another reason for his solitude: the smell. For Widmer had developed a taste for his own excrement, and despite attempts to force him to bathe regularly, could often be found either sitting in or eating it. For the sake of the other patients, he ate his meals alone. It was yet another symptom of his illness. Sadly, human waste was not his only fancy, and his dietary habits included eating lumps of coal or little stones. The coroner blamed the latter delicacy for the diarrhoea that occasioned Widmer's demise in January 1890.

Like many of Broadmoor's foreign legion, Widmer was effectively a refugee who had made his own way in the world. No family or friends ever asked after him, either at Bethlem or Broadmoor. The same was true of the two immigrant men admitted three days after him. The first of these was Yzquierdo, a Spaniard, with straight black hair and Mediterranean looks. He was essentially a terrorist: a member of the Carlist Army, which had fought a guerrilla war in Spain against the establishment. In fear of capture, Yzquierdo had escaped in 1853 to England, the Carlists' ally, where he had begun to forage a basic existence by begging and theft. He was now a vagrant with no fixed abode or place in society.

Only a few weeks after he arrived in his new country, Yzquierdo had tramped to the north of London, to a small rural parish near St Albans. Here, in a field, he encountered the 14-year-old son of a local gamekeeper, who pointed a gun at him and told Yzquierdo forcefully that he was trespassing on the squire's estate. Yzquierdo beat the boy to death with a stick. Taken into custody, he spoke freely at first in Spanish, and a little in English, before he became mute to the world. He stayed silent and awaiting trial for nearly a year, while both the judiciary and the Spanish

Embassy argued over whether he was fit to stand. Considering his background, the result was not entirely surprising. Eventually, he was tried, found guilty and sentenced to death. What was unexpected was the fervour with which the locals were reluctant to see 'the ignorant foreigner' hang, and as a result of their plea for mercy Yzquierdo's sentence was commuted to life imprisonment. Still mute, he was removed to Bethlem.

By the time Yzquierdo arrived in Broadmoor, his refusal to speak had become the norm from which he was prepared to deviate occasionally, if he felt inclined to do so. These inclinations had some sympathy with Widmer's predicament, for Yzquierdo's experience in Southwark had been similar, but with one important difference: Yzquierdo had the company of another Spanish speaker amongst the patients and as a result he had someone to talk to. This companionship was lost when he was moved to Berkshire, and so Yzquierdo became silent again until the arrival of medical officer John Baldwin Isaac in 1875. Isaac spoke a little Spanish, and for ten years he was in daily conversation with Yzquierdo. After Isaac moved on to another job in the hospital, Yzquierdo spoke mostly to himself.

The medical observations on Yzquierdo provide a clue as to what may have happened to him in custody to change his character. He was described as paralysed on the right side, with a lopsided face. He had limited movement, and though he was able to dress himself, he could not wash unaided. Perhaps Yzquierdo had suffered a stroke at some point while he was in Hertfordshire, and this had also affected his speech.

Like Widmer, Yzquierdo was not one of the easiest patients in the asylum to manage. He had a penchant for stealing food and tobacco and was subject to manic phases when he would lash out at those around him. He too spent most of his time at Broadmoor in the back blocks. It was a lonely and helpless existence, and he led it for decades, until he was well into his eighties. Day after day, Yzquierdo ate his meals in silence and stood apart from the other groups in the block's airing court. When Yzquierdo died after nearly 50 years of confinement the event was marked by no one.

One of Yzquierdo's companions on his transfer from Bethlem had been a gentleman named John Flinn, a sailor in his mid-thirties. He was also the first black man to find himself inside the asylum.

Flinn had spent his working life as a crewman, traversing the globe in merchant vessels, including one particular trip to Liverpool in 1855 on a boat from the East Indies. Flinn had been caught housebreaking by the River Mersey and sent to the city's prison at Kirkdale. He would have stayed there and been released in due course had it not been for his unruly and unusual behaviour, which had seen him moved to the local asylum at Rainhill. While a patient there, he attacked a fellow lunatic who died from the effect of Flinn's blows. Like Dadd, Flinn was considered too unfit even to plead in court, and instead he was sent on to Bethlem. There his moods alternated between violence towards all and sundry and deference to the gas lamps in the ward: 'When the gas is lit in the evening he talks to it and treats it with reverence, indeed he worships it'.

Flinn's experience of Broadmoor was as an incurable patient. Spending his time muttering unintelligibly, he was never gainfully employed in any task nor moved beyond the refractory wards. Instead, he worked up a routine as an exhibitionist. He had a propensity first to shred his clothes, then arrange them neatly into a little pile before striding around Block 1 completely naked. The act was a microcosm of Flinn himself: very neat and particular in all his habits, a clean and ordered man in many ways, but unpredictable and impossible to fathom. Like Yzquierdo, he was largely left to his own devices. Flinn died from old age just a few months after the Spaniard.

None of these patients' stories offer any elements of redemption, though the last overseas patient to be brought across from Bethlem demonstrated a little more tractability. William Stolzer had settled in England and was an established member of London's German *émigré* community. Though he had no family, he worked as a bootmaker in and around Regent Street and spoke enough English to get through day-to-day life. All was well for at least four years, before he began to exhibit irrational behaviour. At first he was afflicted only by odd sayings and sudden movements. Then in 1843 he stabbed his fellow worker Peter Heim in the belly with a cobbler's knife. Only Heim's thick, leather apron prevented his death being instant, and he suffered much before he died two days later.

Amongst his colleagues, Stolzer was widely known as being mentally unpredictable. There was a stream of evidence at his trial, though not from medical men, that he was of unsound mind. So it was something of a surprise when the death penalty was passed upon him, and Stolzer was taken off to Millbank to await the noose. Fortunately his counsel was given leave to refer the sentence on to the Home Secretary, who agreed that death seemed an inappropriate penalty, and commuted Stolzer's sentence to one of transportation for life. Stolzer avoided that by acting so strangely that he was given over to Bethlem instead.

A pale, blue-eyed German with dark brown hair, Stolzer became another silent patient in the London asylum despite his grasp of English. Muteness became him. It was clear that he understood conversation, because he could follow instructions to the letter, yet he chose never to engage with his guardians. Rather, Stolzer would make animal, incoherent noises, shouting and screaming, particularly at night. He carried this behaviour through to Broadmoor, though the calming effect of the modern asylum brought about a little change in him. He adjusted to his surroundings enough to become a useful worker on the wards of Block 4, helping to clean the floors and make the beds. It was basic work, but it kept him occupied and seemed to make him happy. And he was not completely lost to the world outside the walls, for he was visited occasionally by some of the German shoemakers that he had left behind in London, even as he lay dying of pneumonia in the summer of 1892.

* * *

Stolzer's experience spoke of the support network of fellow countrymen available to some new immigrants. For most incomers were not like Minor, moneyed and at leisure. They needed to seek out their own kind and find gainful employment, so they gravitated towards familiar accents for survival.

Jacob Schneur was one such incomer. A Russian who had grown up in St Petersburg, Schneur had been forced to flee his birthplace at the age of 40, after becoming wanted in connection with an unfortunate counterfeiting escapade. On the run, and found guilty by the Russian courts in his absence, he took off first to Germany, then France, and in 1865 to London, where he set himself up as a businessman specialising in currency exchange.

Schneur's financial expertise found a ready market. In the nineteenth century, if you wanted to change currencies, then you needed a bill of exchange. There was money to be had from these instruments, and speculators were always on hand to take a bet on whether a bill would bring them profit. If Schneur had intended to go straight, then he may have enjoyed a prosperous City life. Unfortunately, going straight was not exactly what Schneur had in mind. All his counterfeit printing plates had come with him, and it was not long before he had put his energies once again into the very literal pursuit of making money. He acquainted himself with merchants who imported Russian goods and then he printed false bills in roubles, which he swapped for sterling bills and drafts from those same merchants. His deception worked and, emboldened by his success, the next item to arrive hot off his presses were a large number of forged five rouble notes, small enough to be traded directly in exchange for cash. Schneur now had a regular supply of money to meet his monthly outgoings.

However, it was inevitable that he would be found out. It was not long before one of his victims sent an accumulation of the funny money to Schneur's old home town, asking his agent to make an exchange for sterling in St Petersburg at a more favourable price. One day the merchant opened the post to find his roubles returned with the word 'fake' applied to them. He realised that he had been conned, visited the Metropolitan Police and gave them Schneur's address. It was too late, of course: Schneur knew that the net was closing, and he had already left for Paris. Like Dadd, Schneur was arrested in France, extradited, and a short time later he was in Millbank, serving the first of seven years' imprisonment.

No evidence had been produced at Schneur's trial that he was suffering from mental illness and he was treated like a common criminal. However, within a year of his conviction, Schneur was confidently asserting that he was King of Tartary and that he could talk to sparrows. A story also emerged that Schneur was in the habit of writing to the Russian government to inform them of a counterfeiting plot in London, and offering his help to solve it. All he needed, he suggested, was access to lots of money that he could borrow to bait his trap. It was a scheme so transparent that its author was either very stupid, very manipulative or delusionally unaware, as the Home Office concluded. Despite the Millbank governor's view that Schneur was faking it, his prisoner became a patient at Broadmoor in March 1868.

It is difficult not to sympathise with the Millbank governor. Schneur was certainly prone to flights of grandeur, believing himself to be possessed of vast properties in Russia, and that his family held positions of great influence in the Imperial household. He also appeared to be suffering from an imagined persecution; he would grimace in pain, convinced that he was afflicted by some form of wasting disease, forcing himself to vomit in the doctors' presence. Yet at the same time, this ostensibly insane man was highly articulate, writing long letters in English and Russian – usually demanding his discharge – and speaking fluent English and German to anyone who would listen on the ward. He even drew up an essay entitled 'Suggestions for the better management of Broadmoor asylum', which he submitted to William Orange for consideration. Orange's reaction is not recorded, but a tolerant resignation to his charge's views seems most likely. Schneur also objected in writing to the noisier lunatics with whom he initially shared space in Block 3, and petitioned successfully to be moved to the more peaceful Block 5.

This type of strategising did not really fit the behaviour of a mad man. Rather, the doctors described Schneur as 'vain and cunning', and 'attempting to deceive in order to gain his discharge'. Orange quickly grew tired of the endless correspondence with his patient, and by the end of 1870 had managed to establish contact with Schneur's son, who indicated a willingness to look after his father. Rather than send the Russian back to jail, Orange arranged what was effectively a deportation. Schneur was discharged to a Frenchman of Russian extraction who lived in Soho, and was also a friend of one of Schneur's business contacts. This gentleman then holed up the forger in a Charing Cross hotel while he organised a French passport, whereupon Schneur departed once more for the continent, never to darken these shores again.

Schneur is but one example of a Victorian confidence trickster. Another was Jehanger Fearoz, a serial chancer who arrived in London from Bombay in the mid-1870s. Fearoz had gone bankrupt a grand total of four times, but this did not dissuade him from renting a succession of offices in the City, where he posed as an East India merchant. His modus operandi was similar to Schneur's. Fearoz and his English partner, Archibald Hunter, ingratiated themselves with legitimate merchants and then obtained money from them by deception. They would pay a small deposit on goods for order, then intercept the receipts for them at the dock side and use those as collateral to raise further money, disappearing before their original creditors could make them pay the balance on their purchase. It was a routine that had served Fearoz well for years, and allowed him to support his wife and children back home in Bombay and also to keep another home in Maida Vale, where he lived with a young lady by the name of Lily.

Eventually, Fearoz and Hunter were undone by an order for 14 prams placed with the Midland Perambulator Company, for which they had no intention of paying. This so incensed the Midland Perambulator Company that they began asking questions round the London docklands. Fearoz and Hunter were each given four years by the Old Bailey. By this time Fearoz was 52, grey around the temples and his thick moustache. It was rather late in life to begin one's prison career, and the jails he was sent to were not soft options. First he was placed in Wormwood Scrubs, where he was beaten if he misbehaved. Then he was moved to Parkhurst, where he began endlessly pacing the floor of his cell, and then hearing voices. He said that he could hear his wife in Bombay screaming as if she was being beaten. Then, when he was placed in the infirmary, he was convinced that the nurse sent to look after him was his old partner Archibald Hunter. A previously rational and intelligent man, Fearoz was gradually experiencing mental decay.

He arrived in Crowthorne in 1895, where he saw out the remainder of his prison sentence in Block 6. Under medical observation, not only was it clear that his delusions were increasing, but also that his body was riddled with muscular ticks and tremors. The diagnosis was immediate: Fearoz had syphilis, and it had reached the tertiary stage where the disease attacks the workings of the brain. There was no cure. Fearoz's story was only going to end one way. Fourteen years later, long after his criminal sentence had expired, he died on a ward of the Birmingham Borough Asylum.

Fearoz held a slightly different place in British society to the European immigrants. A Parsee of Iranian descent, he was considered as much a part of the British Empire as any other national from one of Victoria's colonies. This meant that he had only ever been under a British jurisdiction and government. There was no consulate or embassy to become involved in his case nor, as for Schneur, an obvious route to deportation. Fearoz was deprived, for the diplomats were often prepared to intercede for patients. To a certain extent they expected it. The Russian Consulate wrote wearily to Orange in 1880 that there was a 'legion of persons who leave our country and take refuge on the hospitable shores of Great Britain', implying that the bureaucrats were ready to deal with the inevitable small percentage of waifs and strays who got into difficulty.

The consulate's letter to Orange had been occasioned by the case of David Salewskam. A man in his mid-twenties, he had been found kneeling in the street in Bow and taken to the City of London Workhouse. Once there he had recovered, only to enter into a state of religious mania, praying, crossing himself, and explaining that he had been sent from heaven. The next afternoon, the nursing staff heard a commotion coming from the ward where Salewskam had been placed. When the medical officer arrived, he found Salewskam brandishing a chair, and the body of a Polish tailor called Harris lying on the floor. Blood, bone and parts of Harris's brain were strewn around the room. Fetching help, the medical staff managed to overpower Salewskam and then strap him to a bed, whereupon he succeeded in knocking out six of his own teeth with the padlock used to secure the straps.

Salewskam was quickly sent to Broadmoor with his arms fastened to his sides and his legs fettered, his skin raw from where his constant movement chafed against his bonds. Three men were required when Salewskam was passed his meals. Left alone in his room with only a rubber chamber pot, a mattress and a sheet to clothe him, Salewskam prowled about his room naked and drinking his own urine.

Orange wrote to the Russian Consulate to ask for an interpreter so that he could try and ascertain his patient's state of mind. Incredibly, the consulate replied that they may not be able to assist: only one of their staff could actually speak Russian, though they could recommend a private contractor instead. Orange took them up on their offer, though to little beneficial effect. 'No information could be got from patient', he wrote. 'Constant delirium and great violence.' So it continued, though with calmer interludes, until Salewskam decided to eat a clay tobacco pipe. It perforated his large intestine.

* * *

No one nation state can be said to have let loose a deluge of lunatics upon the shores of Britain, although most were European, as might be expected by the amount of time and effort that it took to emigrate. Travelling vast distances was not a quick or comfortable proposition and usually immigration had a financial motive. That it happened at all was testament to the success of the national economy. The Broadmoor band of brothers took the step of crossing the seas in the belief that if the streets of England were not paved with gold, they were at least paved with opportunities. Yet the correlation between distance travelled and admission numbers does not quite tally in the asylum. There were just two Frenchman admitted in the Victorian era, for example (and only one other Russian after David Salewskam), and it was very rare for two citizens of the same country to be treated at the same time. Nevertheless, one country was clearly the highest exporter to Victorian Broadmoor: Italy.

Even then, only seven Italian names are entered in Broadmoor's admissions register before the turn of the twentieth century. Sometimes they came and went so quickly that it is unlikely anyone paid them much attention and one of them, Joseph Cerini, holds what may be the record for the hospital's shortest stay: a two-day stopover en route to the Hanwell Asylum in 1868.

Cerini was not the first Italian to visit Crowthorne; that honour goes to Francisco Moretti, a native of Lombardy. The story of how Moretti ended up in Broadmoor began on the shores of Lake Como, where he was born into a small village community. A short man, sporting jet black hair and an olive complexion, at 18 Moretti was provided by his family with the means of moving to London. Obviously a bright and capable young man, he leased a sweet shop in Hackney and soon was making a success of his chosen trade. Business was good: so good in fact that a second shop was leased and opened. Moretti had developed prospects. He was driven, solvent and in control – quite a catch. He fell in love and within two months courted and married his new sweetheart, Elizabeth.

After his marriage things began to go wrong for Moretti. His expanding business was suffering from growing pains, and his cash flow began to be diverted from his own pockets to those of his creditors. The money was drying up and in a short space of time he had lost £100. Moretti could not understand what was happening. At first, he accused his customers of robbing him. When he could find no proof, he dug in his garden, hoping to uncover his missing coins. He banged on the tills of the shops at night in the hope that he could conjure up a spell and magic back some capital. Then, when these methods failed, he began to believe that his own, dear wife was responsible for the losses. He confronted her and they rowed, shouting at each other before the customers. Everything was falling apart, and there appeared to be only one way forward. At dawn the next morning, Moretti took a razor to Elizabeth's throat and then a kitchen knife to his own. The poor woman woke to find her husband standing over her with the blade, jumped from the bedroom window and was rescued by her neighbours as she staggered naked and bleeding around her garden. Neither wound that Moretti inflicted was fatal, but both were severe. His wife's windpipe was torn to such an extent that she was forced to have a tracheotomy tube fitted, and she never recovered fully, dying a year later from her injuries. Her husband bandaged his own wound, and was found insane at trial on the basis of his paranoia. He came to Berkshire in August 1865.

Moretti was young, quiet, orderly and biddable, and was immediately given the privilege of working in the tailor's shop. He was also sent straight to the parole Block 2 as a patient who was no danger to himself or others. Moretti's only visible sign of illness was his devout Catholicism, which he suspected had been a great source of resentment from his wife and others. At Broadmoor, he was deliberately placed on a ward with two other practitioners of the same faith to comfort him.

Unlike many of the international brigade, Moretti had a wide circle of well-wishers who did not forget about him. Relatives of the now deceased Mrs Moretti visited the young man, indicating that they were prepared to forgive, even if they could not forget his actions. Moretti's own brother, also living in London, promised that his family would provide a home for Moretti if he could be returned to Italy. When coupled with Moretti's own industrious and rational behaviour, the offer from this 'respectable man' to care for his sibling pointed to a possible discharge. Everyone was content that Moretti was no danger to anyone, as long as he had companionship and rather less monetary responsibility. After a suitable period of time had elapsed since his trial Dr Meyer, then superintendent, made contact with the Italian Consulate and arranged the practicalities of Moretti's return home. He was escorted by train to the consulate on 8 February 1870, and from there onto the Millwall Docks, where he boarded the steamer *Maria Da Novaro* and left the Thames Estuary bound for Genoa and his friends near Lake Como.

Moretti left one friend behind. For most of the previous two years, he had taken a daily hundred metre stroll across the terrace from Block 2 to Block 5 to converse with a fellow countryman. The two had met at chapel, and would spend the afternoons discussing religion and other matters together in Italian, while the other residents of the Block 5 day room read their newspapers or played games. Moretti was always the visitor, for while his domicile in Block 2 allowed him certain freedoms, patients in Block 5 were not quite parole standard. So after lunch Vincenzo Visoni, a labourer in his mid-fifties, would wait for the crunch of footsteps on the gravel and the sight of Moretti's jet black hair, before another afternoon of conversation would begin. That this was tolerated was testament to the belief that interaction would be of benefit to both men.

Visoni did not share Moretti's stereotypical Italian complexion. He was pale-skinned, with greying hair and sky blue eyes. His looks had contributed to his illness, for Visoni's appearance, as well as his Catholicism, led him to believe that many people labelled him as Irish. In a period of heightened Home Rule nationalism, to be considered Irish could be a problem. Even at Broadmoor on more than one occasion Visoni was moved for his own safety away from patients who had served in the forces and objected to this seemingly republican presence on their ward.

Visoni felt himself a persecuted Fenian for years. Before Broadmoor, work had dried up and he had found accommodation at the parish workhouse of St George in Hanover Square. For four years he had stayed there until his life had been made intolerable by the constant suspicion with which he was treated. No matter how much he tried to convince those around him of his true nationality, he was treated as a terrorist. Desperate for help, one Sunday Visoni had walked to the Italian Consulate in Cheapside, where he paced up and down as he waited for the doors to open. It would have been a long wait, as the consulate was closed for the day. A policeman spotted him and asked Visoni what was going on here, then, and Visoni had responded in robust language suggesting that the policeman should go away. In Visoni's mind, he was accused of being a thief. Somewhat roused, the constable attempted to arrest him, whereupon Visoni reached into his coat pocket and produced a knife. Whether there was any intent to use it was another matter, but brandishing a knife at a member of the Metropolitan Police was only ever going to get him into trouble. Anxious and fidgety, Visoni was considered unfit to plead when he made it to the Old Bailey in January 1868.

Perhaps Visoni's long and troubled life had given him a horror of authority. He had once been a customs official, a little over halfway down the Italian peninsular, working at the border between the Roman Papal States and the Neapolitan Kingdom of the Two Sicilies. Like Yzquierdo, Visoni had been politicised by war and obliged to take arms when the Bourbons of Sicily opposed King Victor Emmanuel's struggle to unite the new Italy of 1861. Visoni claimed that after the war, he had been incarcerated as a political prisoner, and later forced to leave Italy. Bereft of a country and a livelihood, Visoni had ended up working in London, leaving a wife and three children back in the Mediterranean while he still looked over his shoulder at those who accused him of treachery.

Visoni remained a haunted figure as his delusions transformed. It was not long before he was shouting out and screaming at night, complaining like Minor that he was being attacked and abused. Shrill singing of infamy could be heard in Block 5 in both Italian and French, as Visoni stammered with excitement while he found his words. Sadly, his accusatory behaviour eventually alienated his pal Moretti. When Visoni discovered that his countryman had begun Italian lessons for another patient in Block 5, he took it as a personal infidelity and resolved to have no more to do with him. Moretti left without being able to say goodbye.

That the relationship had been of benefit became apparent when Moretti left. Afterwards, Visoni's mental health deteriorated quickly and he was moved through the blocks from 5 to 4 and then to Block 6, the hidden back block. Once there, although he helped out in the scullery, he refused to ever go outside again. Visoni suffering from both auditory and physical hallucinations. As with so many patients who became aware of electricity, Visoni began to report that powerful electric shocks were delivered to him at night. It was clear that there was no hope of recovery. Thirty-five years of torment later, he died in Broadmoor at the grand old age of 91.

* * *

Without intervention beyond the regime of 'moral treatment' and the occasional sedative or purgative, it was a hit and miss affair as to whether any patient would regain enough health to be discharged, like Moretti, or end up in chronic care like Visoni. The chronic cases would almost certainly die inside an asylum. Even for those who recovered their health, a life outside the asylum was not automatic. The recovery of a rational mind was merely the first prerequisite for discharge, rather than a reason for discharge in itself. Before parole could be recommended, an investigation of its possible outcomes was first required.

This investigation was largely one of risk management and deciding the likelihood of the patient becoming unwell again. Typical factors for consideration were the chances of them encountering their previous triggers for insanity, or whether the patient had a support network beyond the walls to help them navigate their way through life. The last factor was due to the requirement for the 'moral treatment' to be replicated in civilian life. Bed and board, the right environment, routine and work or other industrious occupation all had to be ticked off on the checklist by the superintendent before the Home Office would comply with a request to exit. These conditions tended to place the international patients at a disadvantage, for they were less likely to have close family at hand. A deportation, such as Schneur's or

Moretti's, afforded an alternative in these circumstances, but it was a more complex procedure. As a result, foreign patients who were discharged in the typical fashion were usually those who had become naturalised and put down roots in England.

Even when everything seemed to be in place for a successful discharge, the process was not without risks. Felix Mayer, a watchmaker from Baden in southern Germany, had married an English woman and fathered four children. The couple had made their home in Newbury, only 20 miles from Broadmoor. At the age of 42, Mayer's livelihood failed and he took to drink. Mayer's alcohol-fogged mind led him to doubt those around him, and although for years he had lived as an integrated member of the local community, now he saw his penury as a consequence of prejudice. Increasingly confused, isolated and scared, Mayer set fire to a haystack near Reading as a cry for help.

When he arrived at Broadmoor in 1865, his feelings of persecution extended to the other patients, who he believed were ridiculing him, especially for his work in the asylum shoemaking shop. Mayer's self-esteem had hit rock bottom. He felt that he 'amused himself with a piece of leather', while the other patients did the proper work. These feelings of inferiority gave him headaches. But gradually, Mayer became a happier, model patient. He no longer felt worried, was well-behaved, and worked hard at his shoemaking. Perhaps once away from drink, Mayer detoxed and rediscovered his *joie de vivre*.

Mayer's wife was a regular visitor to the asylum, and when his brother also began to take an interest in him, Dr Orange felt that it might be sensible to raise the question of discharge. Mayer was no longer actively insane, so the prerequisite was met, and further he had people around who cared about him. Mayer himself was also keen to be granted passage back to Newbury.

However, Mayer's discharge on 19 August 1871 was a disaster. Collected by his brother Matthew in the morning, by four o'clock that afternoon he was back at the asylum gatehouse, wild-eyed and in a hopelessly manic state. Almost as soon as he left, while the two men walked the road to Crowthorne Station, Mayer had been overcome by a bleak and futile vision of his future. 'I could see nothing before me but indigence,' he explained. Mayer sat, brooding intently, as the train transported them to Reading. At his brother's terraced house in the west of the town Mayer sat in the back room while lunch was prepared in the kitchen. Something inside him snapped. He stood up and peered round the door. "I cannot face the world again: take me back to Broadmoor," he announced to his startled relatives. They obliged him.

His readmission was an acceptance by the hospital that Mayer would now be unlikely to ever leave. It was rare enough to be discharged once and to be discharged twice would have required some unforeseen improvement in circumstances. When Mayer's wife died the next year there was no longer even a family home for him to return to. At least he was not a burden at Broadmoor. Although he remained profoundly depressed, he was a low risk patient and rejoined the routine as if he had never left his bedroom in Block 2. Once again he took up his slow, steady work in the shoemaking shop, occasionally anxious about his own performance. He died from a stroke in 1878.

Cases such as these always taxed the Home Office, which felt strongly that Broadmoor was not a place that patients should return to purely because they felt safer there than in the outside world. If a patient was rational, as Mayer clearly was, and no danger to society, then they should take their chances on the outside. However, these views were seldom shared by the doctors in charge of the asylum. For them, the whole point of their system of mental health treatment was that their community acted as a refuge for their patients, providing the safe haven that kept them sane. They believed that their duty of care was not extinguished solely by the application of a judicial warrant of conditional discharge. The clinicians usually got their way.

The naturalised patients all tended to share a similar back history to Mayer. Almost entirely men (one German woman was the sole foreign female admission), they had come to Britain as economic migrants, found that they liked it and integrated, often marrying but certainly contributing positively to society for years. They were indistinguishable from the other labourers and tradesmen who made up the bulk of Broadmoor's male population and accepted by them. Only from their accent or their skin colour would any casual observer have guessed that a patient's life might have begun overseas. Even their names did not necessarily provide a clue.

William Brown was a naval pensioner who had settled in Sittingbourne, Kent. Like John Flinn, Brown was a black sailor who came to England through his work. He hailed from Demerara, then part of the British colony of Guyana and squashed against the South American coast by the larger Brazilian Empire. Brown was born overlooking the Atlantic Ocean and in his mid-twenties he decided to follow the horizon and join the British Navy. The navy was good to Brown. Not only did it offer him a career, but in due course it introduced him to his wife, Elizabeth. In 1869, when Brown was 37, the couple met in Sheerness and married two years later. Elizabeth was a widow and she welcomed Brown into her home opposite the town's railway station and adjacent to the dockyard. Brown became stepfather to her children, as well as a father to his own.

By the time Brown retired in 1881 he had served for 21 years, achieved the rank of petty officer first class and received a good conduct medal alongside his pension. In theory, Brown was winding down and looking forward to earning a second income as a labourer and spending more time with his family. But he was becoming increasingly unpredictable, distant and moody. When he and Elizabeth argued about the children, Brown concluded that there was no future for them. Late one winter's night, nearly two years after he retired, Brown took up a hatchet and plunged it into the back of Elizabeth's head. As she lay unconscious on the bedroom floor he first cut her throat and then his own, before staggering downstairs and setting a fire under the stairs. Fortunately, the noise woke the children and Brown's elder stepson was able to raise the alarm, though he suffered a stab wound from the older man for his trouble.

No motive was offered at Brown's trial for his savage attack. There was no evidence of jealousy or infidelity. Obtaining information from Brown himself was difficult, as he had wielded the razor with such gusto that he had severed his own larynx. He sat in the dock throughout proceedings and sucked down air through a rudimentary tracheotomy tube. His defence lawyers were convinced that he was unaware of what he had done. They suggested that Brown had suffered a blackout, possibly caused by an epileptic fit. The jury took 45 minutes to declare him insane.

Brown's time at Broadmoor was short. Though he could hardly speak, he was obviously devastated at the realisation of what he had done. He wept and asked to be allowed to go on his own 'long journey', that he might die and find forgiveness from God. By the end of March 1885, he was bedridden with pleurisy. He died three months later.

Though his own story had no happy ending, Brown's three young children struggled on. They were not, as the children of patients sometimes were, taken in by friends or relatives. Instead, they were taken by the parish overseers to the Sheppey Union Workhouse and consigned to the orphan ward. But Amanda, Anna and Donald Brown never lost contact with their father. As Donald was sent to school and Amanda was placed in service, it fell to Anna to write to Broadmoor. She was suffering from a degenerative eye condition and so she remained in the care of the workhouse. Anna wrote to her father to tell him what was going on in his children's lives, and she organised visits to see him. Though he had lost his wife, William Brown was not alone at the end.

Brown's children went on to play their own parts in English society. Donald Brown even found his own small place in history. Sent by the workhouse to attend the Greenwich Royal Hospital School, where the orphan sons of sailors were taught a trade, he later followed in his father's footsteps and embarked on a career at sea. He also became a political radical in the East End of London and married a prominent suffragette, Eliza Adelaide Knight. In 1919 he was decorated for single-handedly dragging a pile of burning munitions away from the Woolwich Arsenal, an act that probably saved many lives. Donald Brown might have been the son of a Broadmoor patient, but he became a hero.

* * *

Ex-forces patients were a mainstay of many a Victorian asylum. Wars were a regular part of British life in the nineteenth century, and each temporary outbreak of peace resulted in another demobbed cohort likely to feed the network of hospitals for the insane. By the time that Broadmoor opened, these wars tended to be fought far from our own shores, more often in our theatres of influence instead, and gave foreign soldiers the opportunity to relocate as well. The winds of conflict blew various cases into Crowthorne, for William Brown was not the only patient who had enlisted.

One was surgeon William Chester Minor, of course. Another, more representative old soldier was Major Joseph Pelezarski, a Pole and veteran of the Crimean War. Pelezarski was also a surgeon and had served with the French as part of the coalition of allies seeking to stop Russia's aggression on modern-day Turkey. When the war ended in 1856, Pelezarski arrived in London, where his mental condition degenerated. He took to the streets, unable to provide for himself. He began to receive communications from spirits, who would offer him helpful advice on beatific matters. One suggestion was that to obtain sainthood, he would have to renounce footwear. So Pelezarski began to tramp around barefoot.

His was a classic case of progressive dementia and by this stage the question was merely in what type of institution Pelezarski would end up. Incredibly, instead he found a saviour. Though aged 50, unkempt and shoeless, he did not lack charm, and he was befriended by a Russian woman whose acquaintance he had made. The connection was genuine, and soon the relationship developed. But Pelezarski's voices had not deserted him, and unfortunately they took a dim view of the new direction in his life. Before long his inability to rationalise his physical needs with his spiritual ones had led to domestic violence. At the end of 1860 Pelezarski's neighbours, already suspicious from the bruises on his mistress, were quick to investigate when they heard screams coming from the shared passage outside his rooms.

They found the lady of the house alive, but bleeding from a head wound where Pelezarski had hit her with a board. He was still beside her and both were stark naked. When the other residents appeared Pelezarski ran, but was soon overpowered then restrained until the police arrived. His companion was helped back inside and dressed. Up before the Middlesex Sessions, Pelezarski exhorted crossly that the woman was really very fond of him, and that he only 'beat her because she was naughty'.

Pelezarski ended up in the asylum system: first Bethlem, then Fisherton House in Salisbury, before his transfer to Broadmoor. His appearance at Fisherton, the more low-key government annexe for criminal lunatics, implied a rather harmless case and so he turned out. He felt disinclined to work, but was otherwise well-behaved. He spoke a little English and rather more French, though his preference was to be left to stand alone, with his head drooping towards the floor. Still beset by spirits, he died at the age of 92 in 1904.

Another foreign soldier, Wilhelm Kirchhoff, had served in the Prussian Army in Westphalia. Dark complexioned, with deep hazel eyes and brown hair, Kirchhoff had been an infantryman until at the age of 27, delusions of persecution overwhelmed him and he was taken off to a madhouse.

Kirchhoff's tale bears one similarity with Minor's, as on his discharge from the army in 1857, he decided to travel the world. He sailed across the Atlantic, bound for the United States and a new life. When he arrived he followed what he knew, enlisted in the US Army and attained the rank of corporal. All was well for a while, until his paranoia returned and he quit the army to work on a farm. It was not long before he became convinced that the farmer suspected him of adultery with his wife. So Kirchhoff stole a horse, rode to port and found another ship, this time bound for London.

He had been in England for three years when at Reading, he pointed a loaded pistol against a policeman's temple and threatened to pull the trigger. 'He needs to be watched', wrote Superintendent Meyer. An obsessive character, when he was not making threats or breaking crockery, Kirchhoff compulsively ate or dieted. As a result his weight either ballooned or fell off him, and when he wasn't slimming, he frequently had to be force-fed through a pump. As a diversion, he took up writing to the Queen, never once deterred by the lack of reply.

The modern observer might wonder whether any ex-forces patients had suffered some form of trauma. Kirchhoff's end hints at this possibility. On a summer's night in 1873, when he was 45 years old, Kirchhoff waited until all was quiet in the asylum. He got out of bed, tied one end of his braces round a piece of skirting board and then passed the other end through the ventilation grate high on the wall of his room, knotting the fabric to secure it. Leaving a generous end of the cord free, he took the mattress from his bedstead and placed it on the floor, before turning the frame on its side and resting that on the bedding and against the wall. When he was satisfied that the frame was stable Kirchhoff climbed up this structure, fastened the free end of the braces around his neck as tightly as he could and simply kicked the bed frame over. With his head tethered near the ceiling and the braces held quite taut, the whole process was effortlessly efficient. Kirchhoff dropped a little under three feet, just enough to break his neck cleanly and leave his toes brushing weightlessly against the floor.

* * *

Far away from landlocked Berkshire, ropes were cast off as ships belonging to Victorian merchants swept gracefully from shore to shore. It was an industry as ordered and as organised as the armed forces, yet to be on a merchant ship was to experience their own peculiar environment. Each ship's crew had a rootless life, without the structure or the welfare of the regular navy – a basic and hard existence. As a result, some form of mental self-management was almost a prerequisite for successful seafaring. The realities of a lifetime's sailing also provided a contradictory existence, surrounded as sailors were with a surfeit of outside space, and only the most restricted opportunities for being at large within it. At its claustrophiliac heart, it was the sort of environment where every small act or passing thought could be magnified.

The sea links all the stories of the international brigade, for it was the sea that bought each of them to England. Nor is there a shortage of mariners' tales to add to those already heard: William Hill, a Russian thief; Carl Lillia, a retired Finn found wandering in someone's house; Francesco Poggi, an Italian who stabbed his first mate while their vessel was in Falmouth harbour. These unfortunates did not all register in the local consciousness, though Poggi caused some Cornish consternation as he was kept, raving, in the local two-room gaol for over a month while the Home Office decided whether or not to put him back on board. Eventually the local police chief took Poggi up to Crowthorne himself. The Crown declined to reimburse him for his trouble.

Like so many Broadmoor patients, the stories of these men remain somewhat opaque, and often it is the sailors who came from the farthest flung places that have left the clearest, most evocative biographies. William Thompson is one of them. Born in Charleston, South Carolina in 1831, Thompson's father was English, his mother was German and his English grandfather had had a Native American mistress. He was short but burly, tipping 17 stone, with the broad facial features of a non-European man and the curly, battleship grey hair and beard of a middle-aged one.

In their own small way, the Thompsons had attempted to pursue the American dream. There was a family home in Charleston and another 38 acres of land nearby, purchased with some distant aim of building a homestead. But the settlers' life was still hand-to-mouth and employment a necessity. William was apprenticed to a baker, but ran away when he was 18 to a life at sea, occasionally making port back on the Eastern Seaboard to spend time with his widowed mother.

At the end of one long voyage William Thompson's ship sailed up the Clyde and he arrived in Glasgow. At this point he already had two illegitimate children in distant harbours and the woman he now picked up down by the docks would go on to bear him two more. They married and set up home together in a tenement block. Thompson saved as much as he could, sending some money home to his mother and keeping the rest to support his new family. So far, so stable. But then his wife died, and leaving his children in his mother-in-law's care, he went back to sea.

In the summer of 1880, Thompson was in Hong Kong, en route from Australia, and working on board the steamship *Peru*. He was no longer used to the heat, and he suffered from sunstroke. Thompson was also suffering from drink; he had always been a hard drinker but had begun imbibing to excess. As the *Peru* left port to make for London, it was blown by an ill wind across the Indian Ocean. First the captain became sick, and was confined largely to bed while the crew quarrelled, and then William Thompson became suspicious.

His suspicions began with the food. Even though he was responsible for its preparation, Thompson reckoned that other members of the crew were poisoning it. While the ship tossed and turned on the waves, Thompson sought out the chickens stowed on board, or a pig called Murphy, and had the animals act as his tasters before he felt safe to eat. This kind of behaviour set everyone on edge. When Murphy's snout turned sore, probably due to a porcine cold, Thompson accused one of the crew, Alexander Ogilvy, of poisoning him. Ogilvy swore at Thompson,

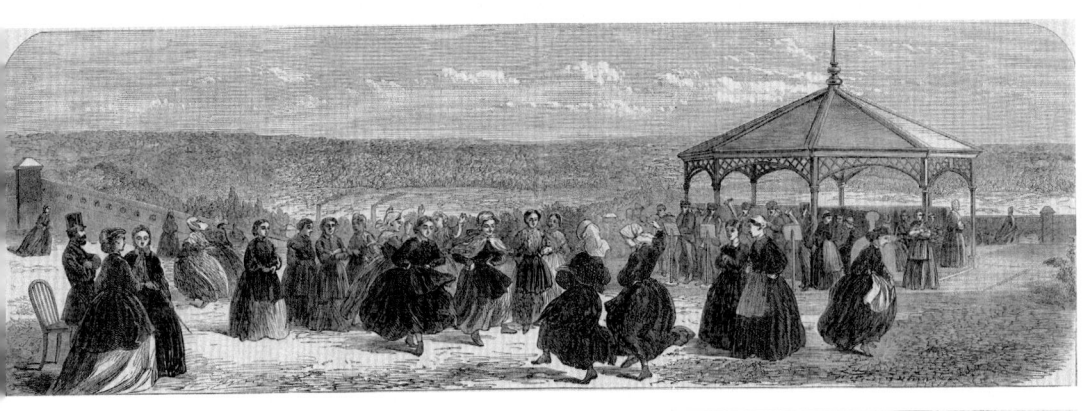

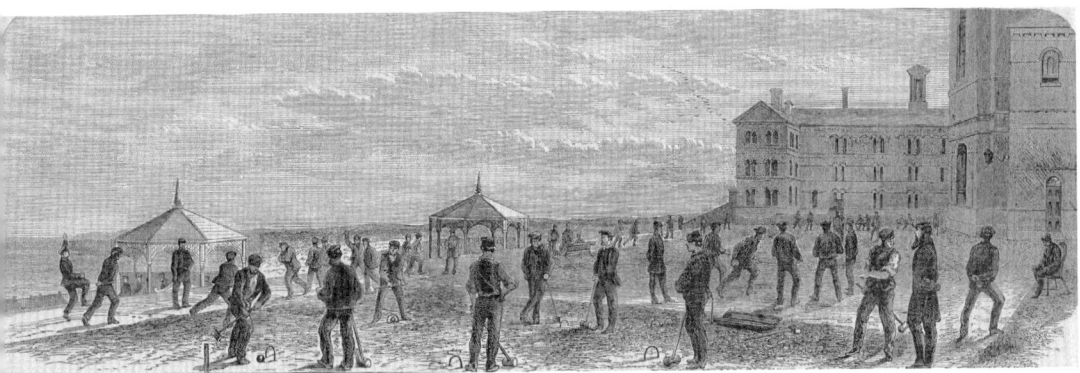

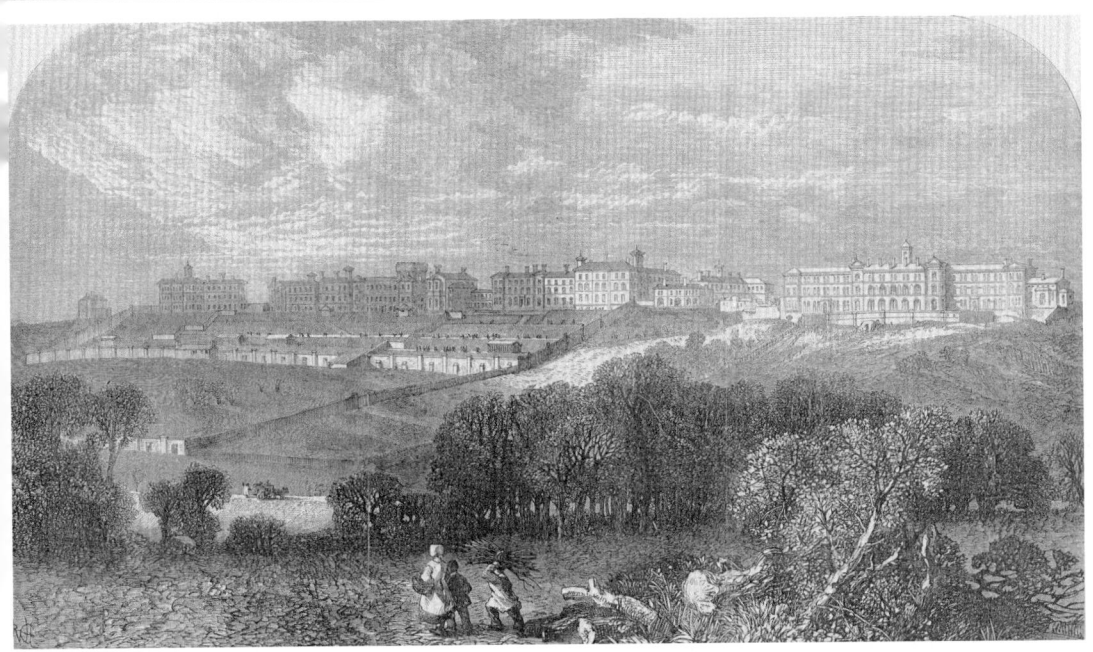

These sketches were published in a voyeuristic feature by the *Illustrated London News* in 1867. (*Top*) The asylum band plays as the women dance and a doctor looks on. (*Centre*) Croquet and cricket are being played on the lawn. (*Bottom*) Panorama from the south. The larger male side is to the left and the female side to the right. (*All reproduced by permission of Reading Libraries*)

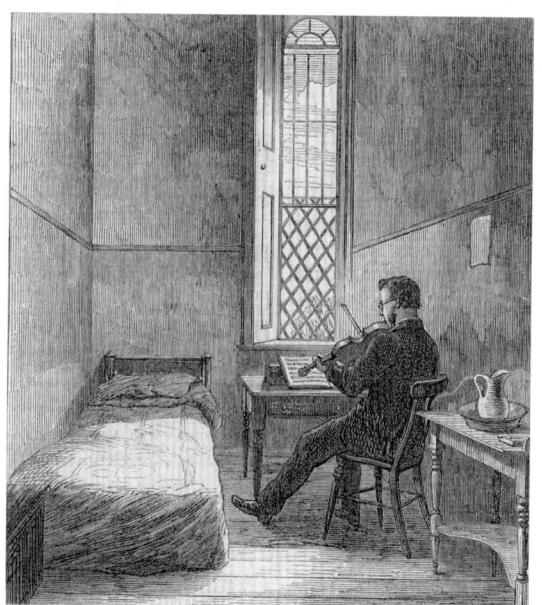

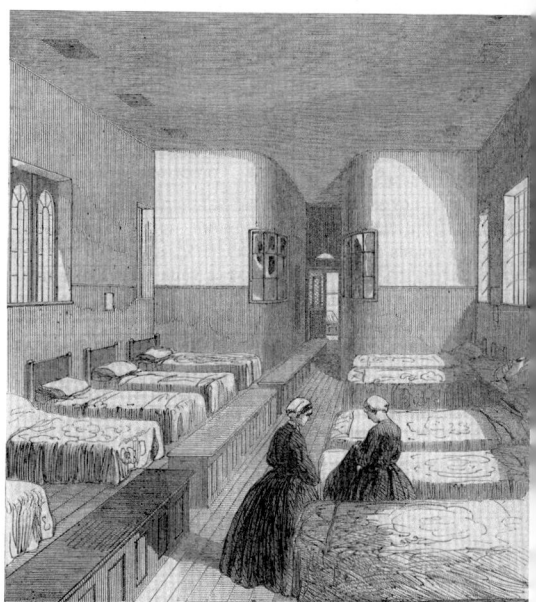

(*Top left*) A patient in Block 2 plays his violin in his bedroom. (*Top right*) In the female dormitory patterned fabric can be glimpsed on the bed linen. One summer visitor to Broadmoor remarked on the brightness of the female wards, with vases of freshly cut flowers in every corridor.
(*Bottom*) A male day room, probably in Block 2. It has been suggested that the bearded figure on the far right is Richard Dadd. (*All reproduced by permission of Reading Libraries*)

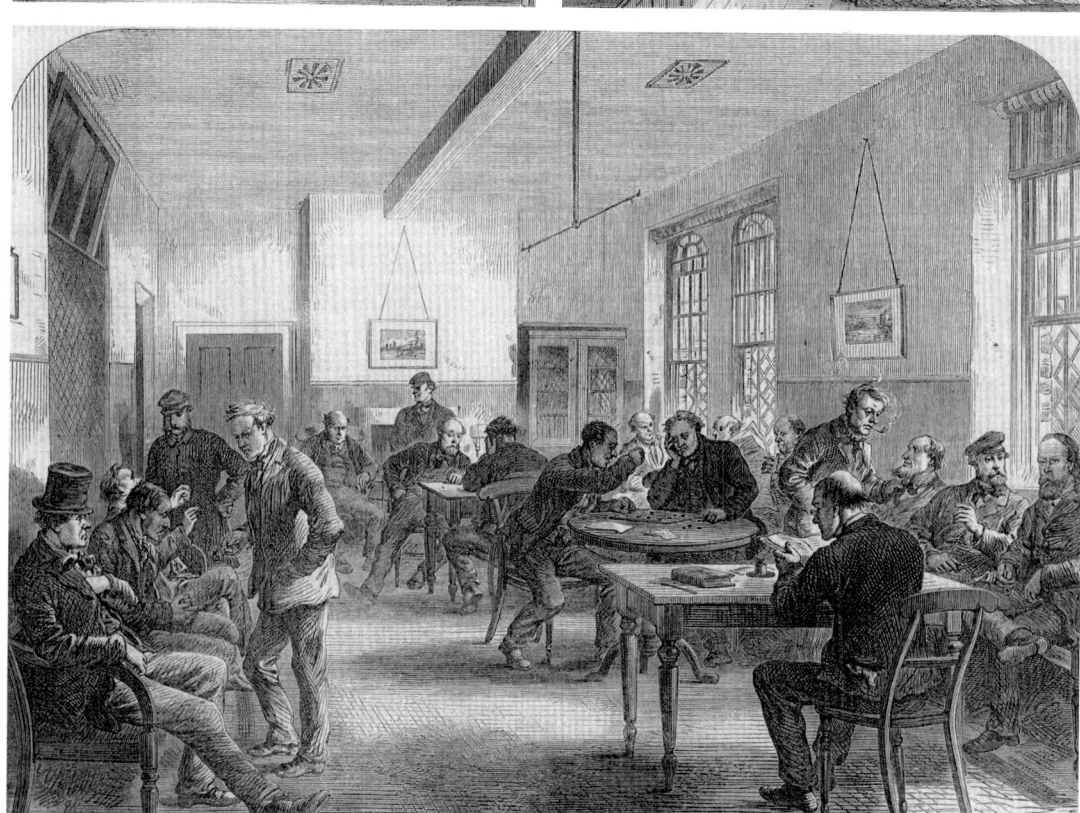

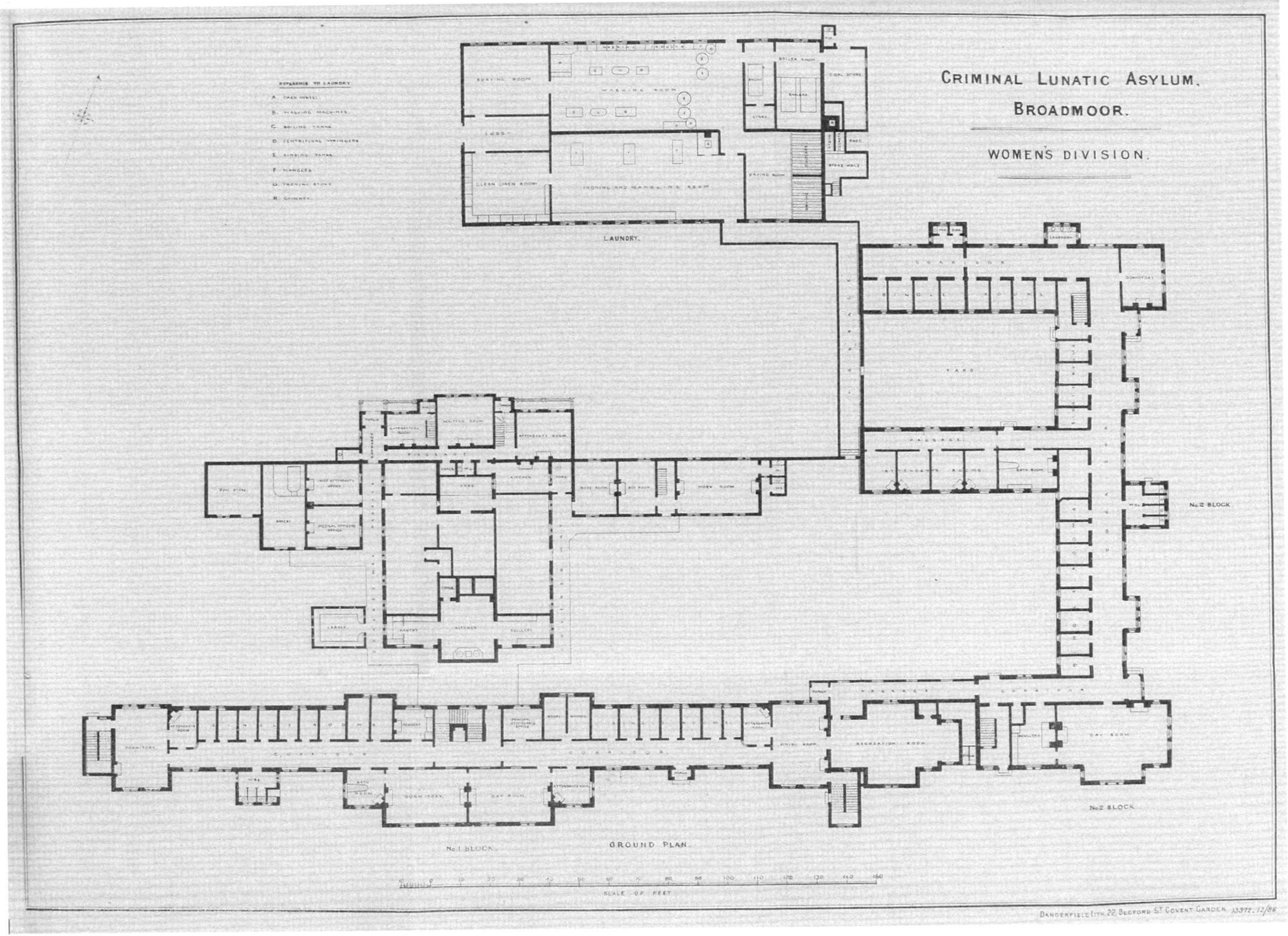

Ground floor plans of the female side in 1885, as laid out at the end of Orange's leadership.
(Reproduced by permission of the Wellcome Library, London)

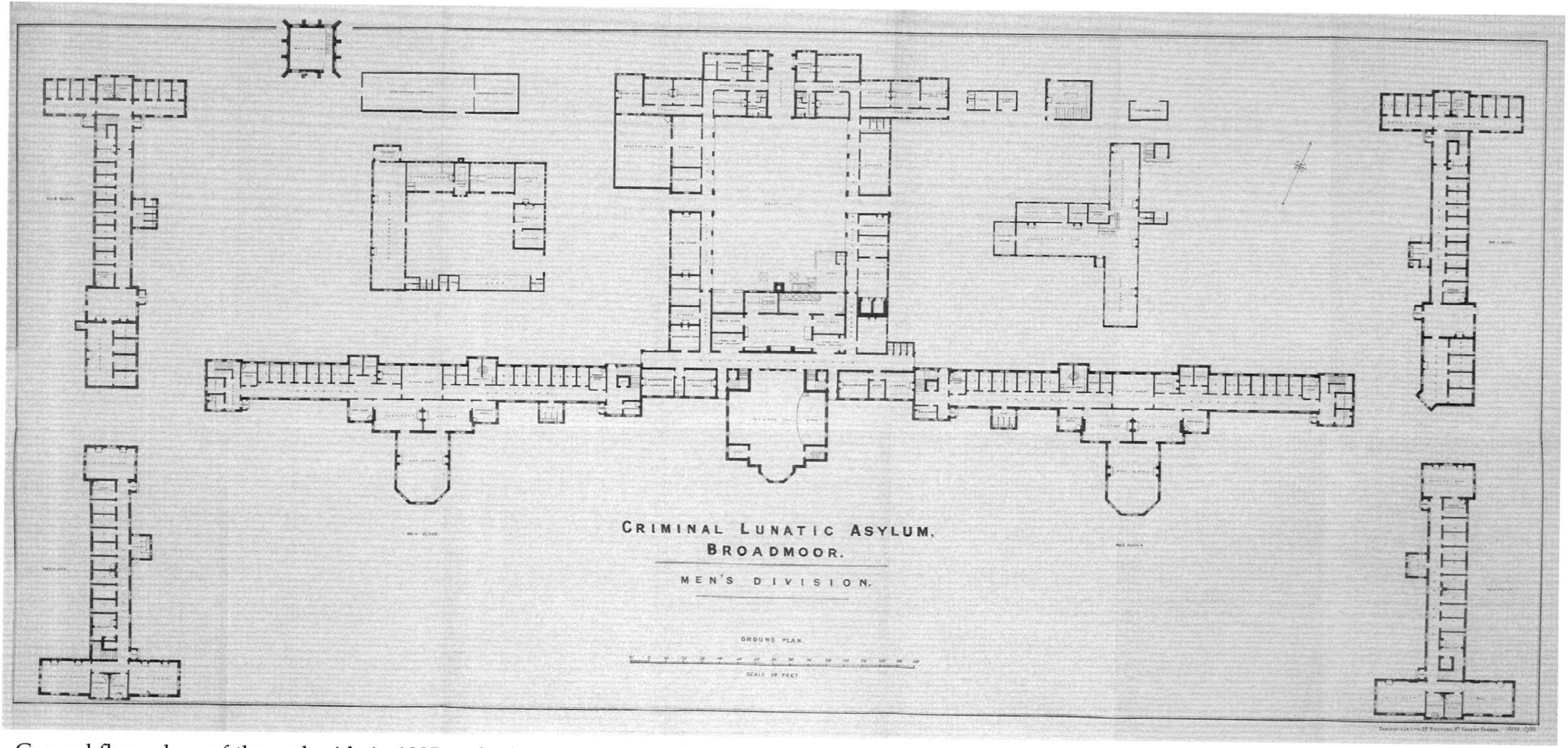

Ground floor plans of the male side in 1885, as laid out at the end of Orange's leadership. *(Reproduced by permission of the Wellcome Library, London)*

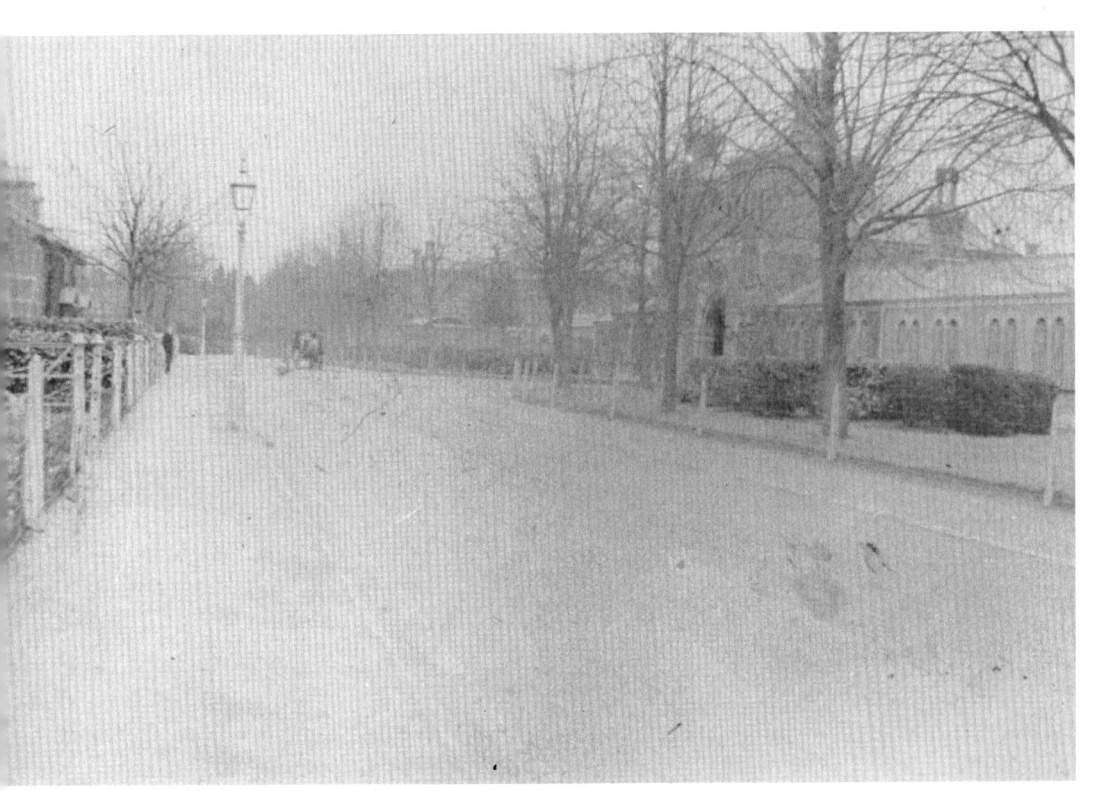

The road to Broadmoor, late nineteenth century. On the left is a row of attendants' cottages, now demolished, while the gatehouse lies behind the trees to the right. The female entrance is further along the road. *(Reproduced by permission of the Berkshire Record Office)*

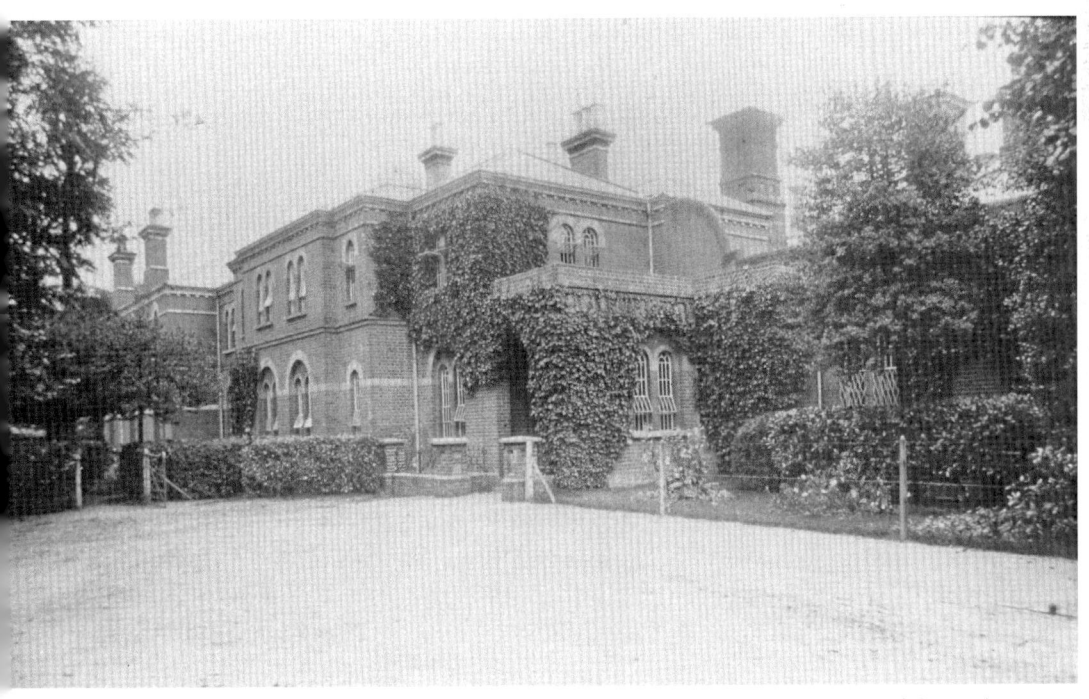

The women's entrance, c.1900. The much less imposing gateway to the female side of the asylum. Though there are bars on the windows, the overall appearance is more of a country house. *(Reproduced by permission of the Berkshire Record Office)*

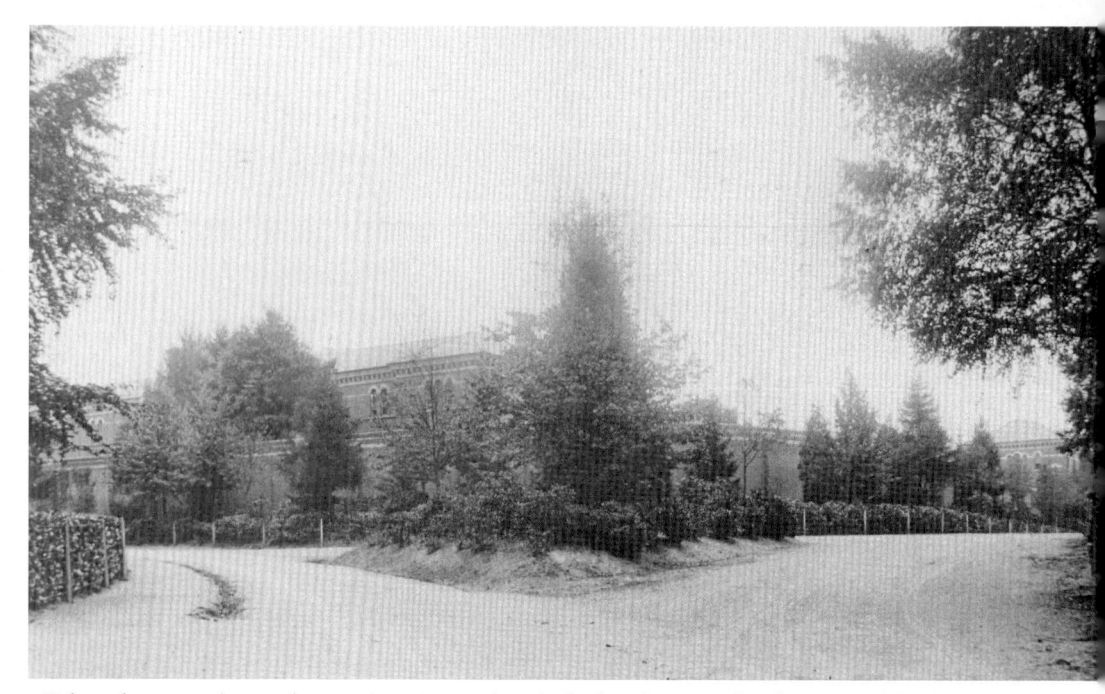

Taken the same day as the previous image (*overleaf*), the photographer has turned back towards the boundary wall on the male side. The road towards the left led to the superintendent's house.
(*Reproduced by permission of the Berkshire Record Office*)

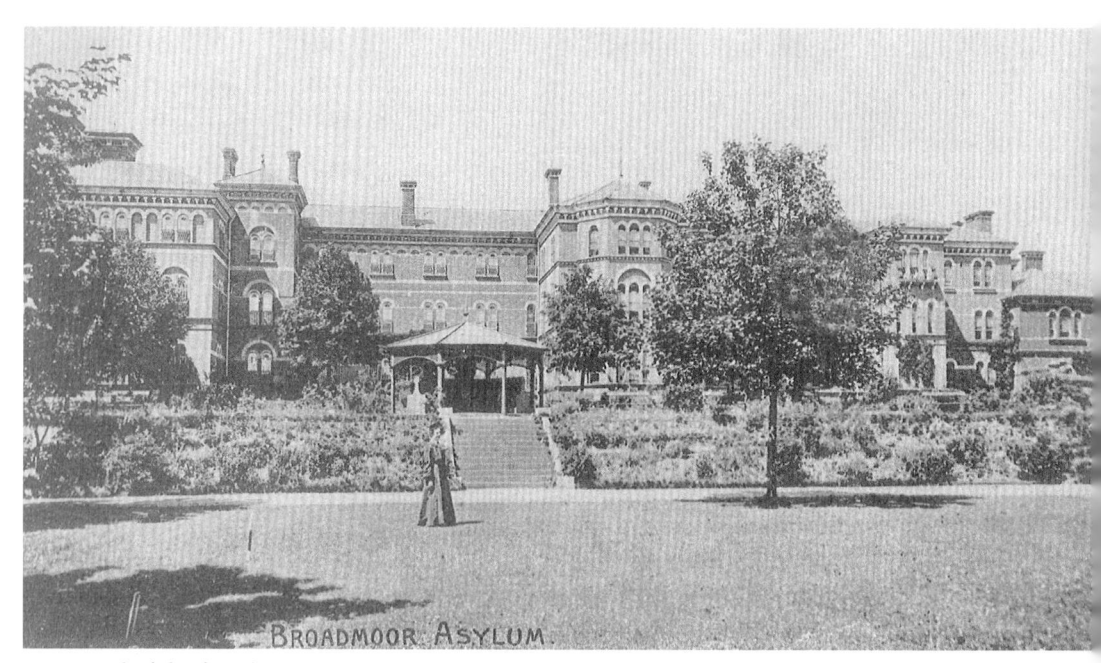

Postcard of the female gardens, c.1900. The south side of the original female block, where the less chronically ill women were accommodated. Croquet hoops are visible on the lawn; the bandstand is behind the solitary, unknown figure.

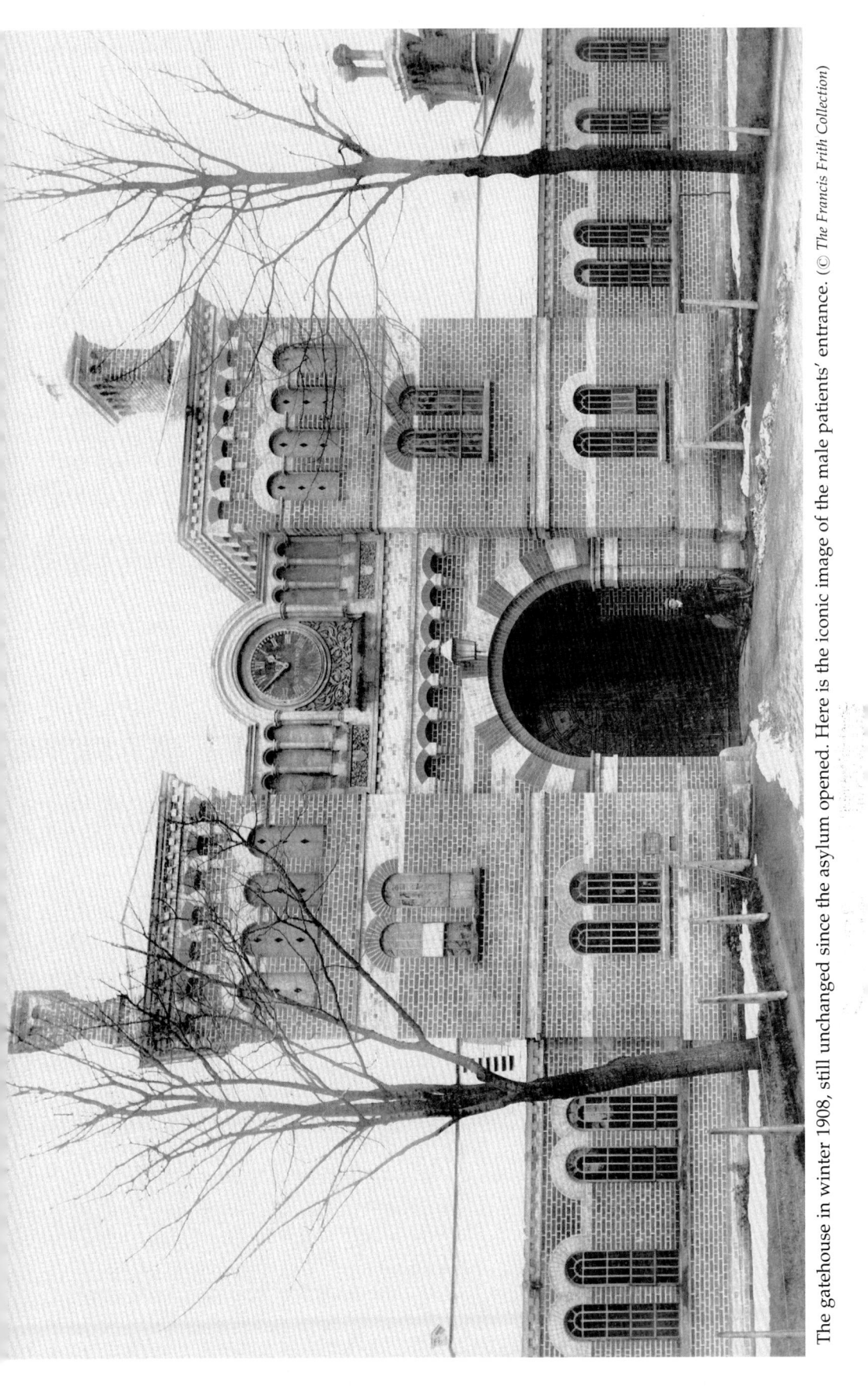

The gatehouse in winter 1908, still unchanged since the asylum opened. Here is the iconic image of the male patients' entrance. (© *The Francis Frith Collection*)

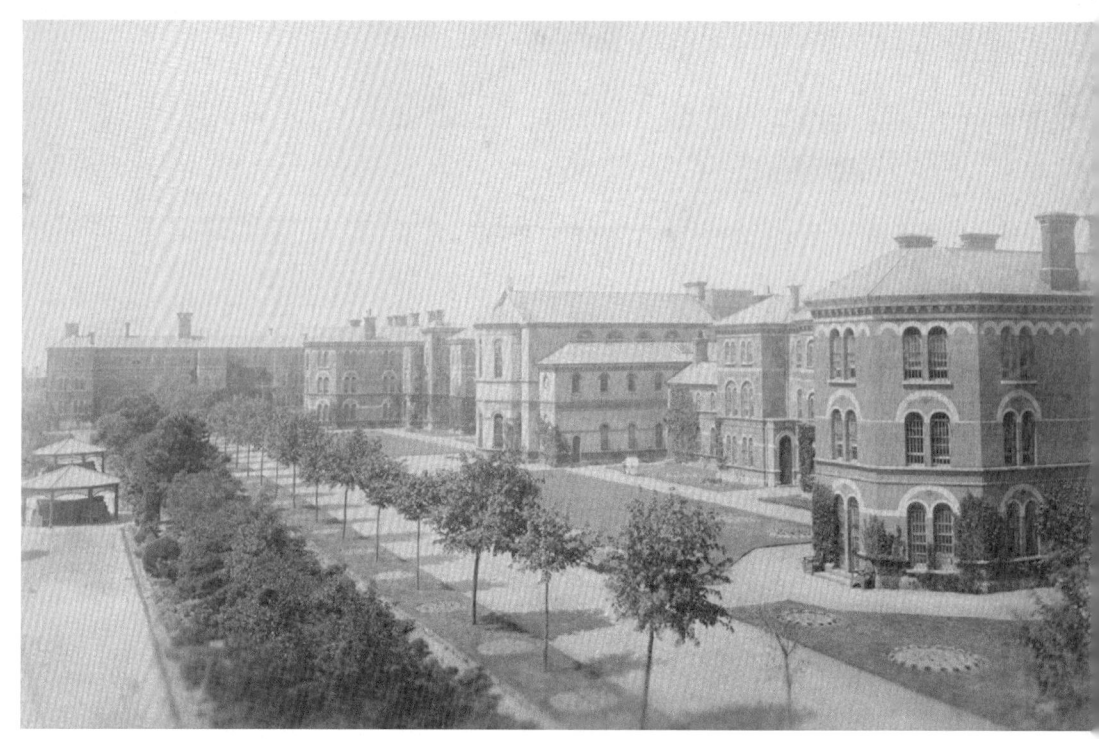

A view across the upper terrace, 1886. This shows the southern range of buildings on the male side as seen from the top floor of Block 2. (L-R) Block 5, Block 4, administrative block (with the central hall and chapel above in lighter brick), Block 3. This photograph was probably taken by a professional photographer for Orange's retirement, as a studio was not established on site until 1899. (*Reproduced by permission of West London Mental Health NHS Trust/Berkshire Record Office*)

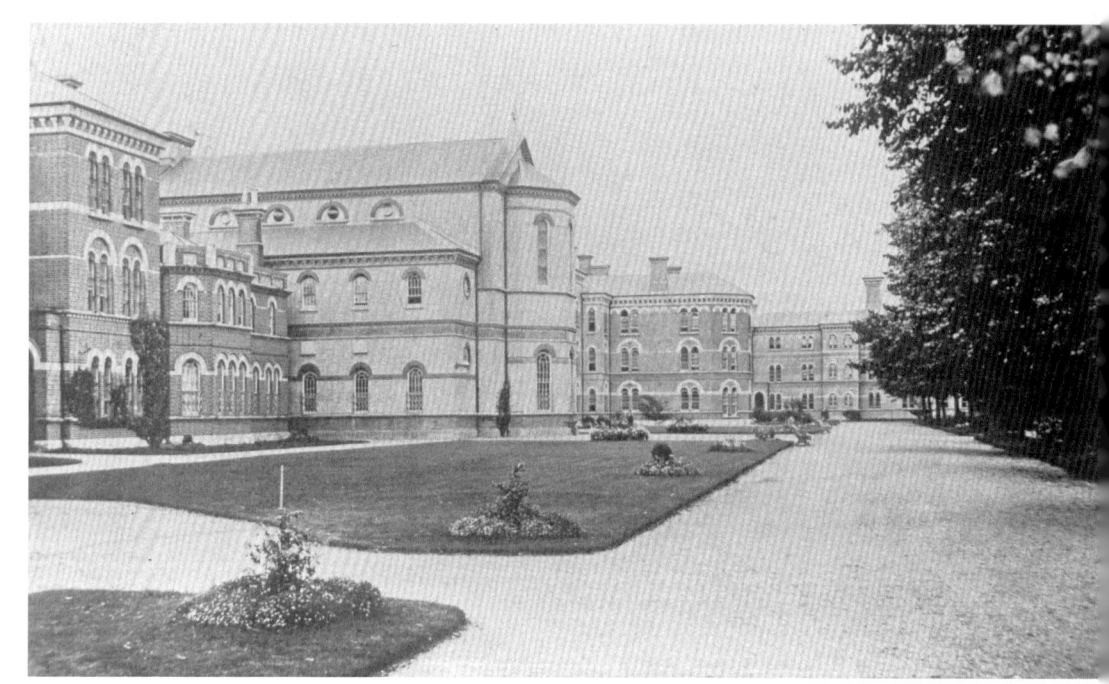

Looking east along the upper terrace, early twentieth century. Taken from the end of Block 4, looking back towards the chapel and Block 3. Block 2 can be seen at the far end of the terrace. (*Reproduced by permission of the Berkshire Record Office*)

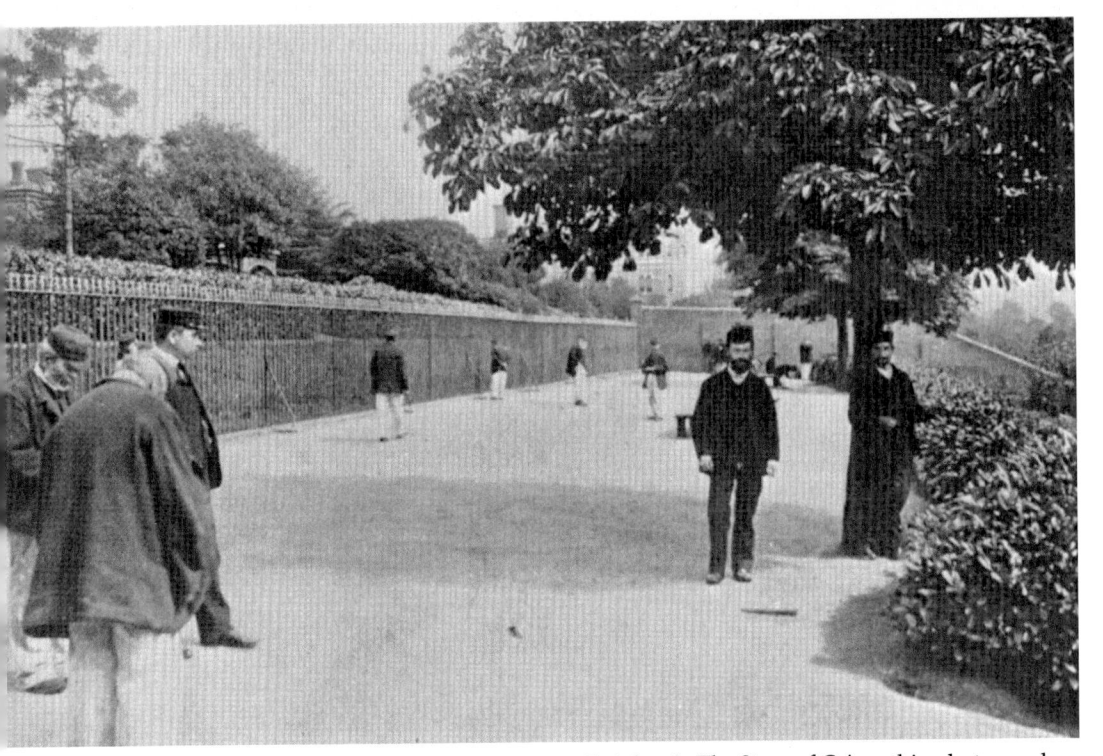

Patients and staff on the terrace, 1908. From Hargrave L Adam's *The Story of Crime*, this photograph looks east across one of the lower terraces, with the edge of Block 2 in the background. Adam, a true crime writer, was shown round Broadmoor with his camera. He reported that many patients absented themselves from the communal areas once they saw him readying his equipment.

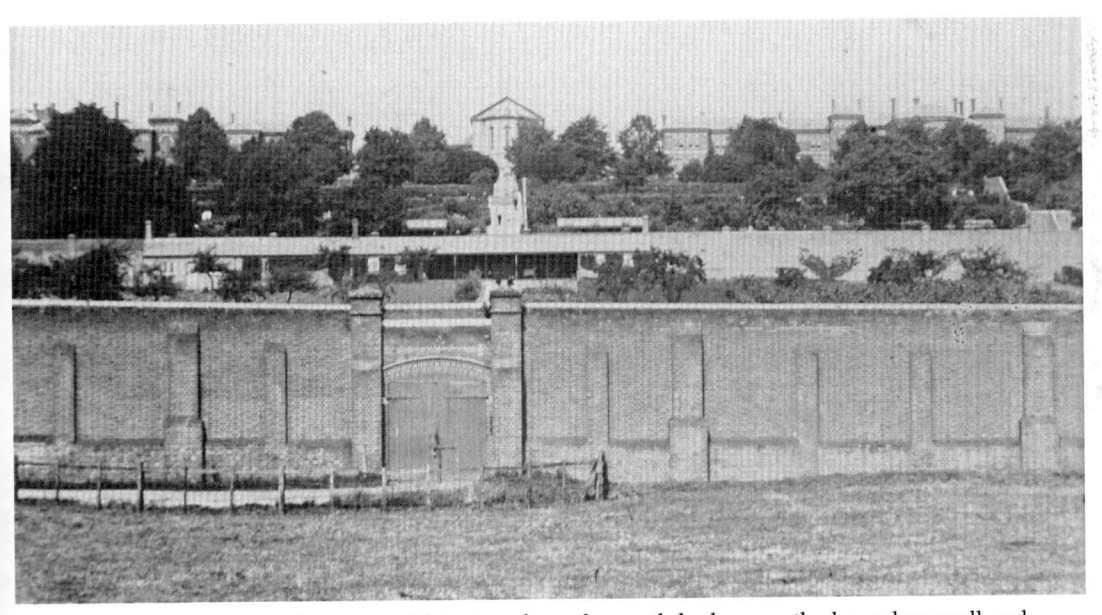

The terrace, early twentieth century. This view from the south looks over the boundary wall and gives a clear view of the terrace. The chapel can be seen in the centre distance. Immediately beyond this boundary were parts of the farm and the cricket pitch. The doorway allowed working parties out into the wider estate. (*Reproduced by permission of the Berkshire Record Office*)

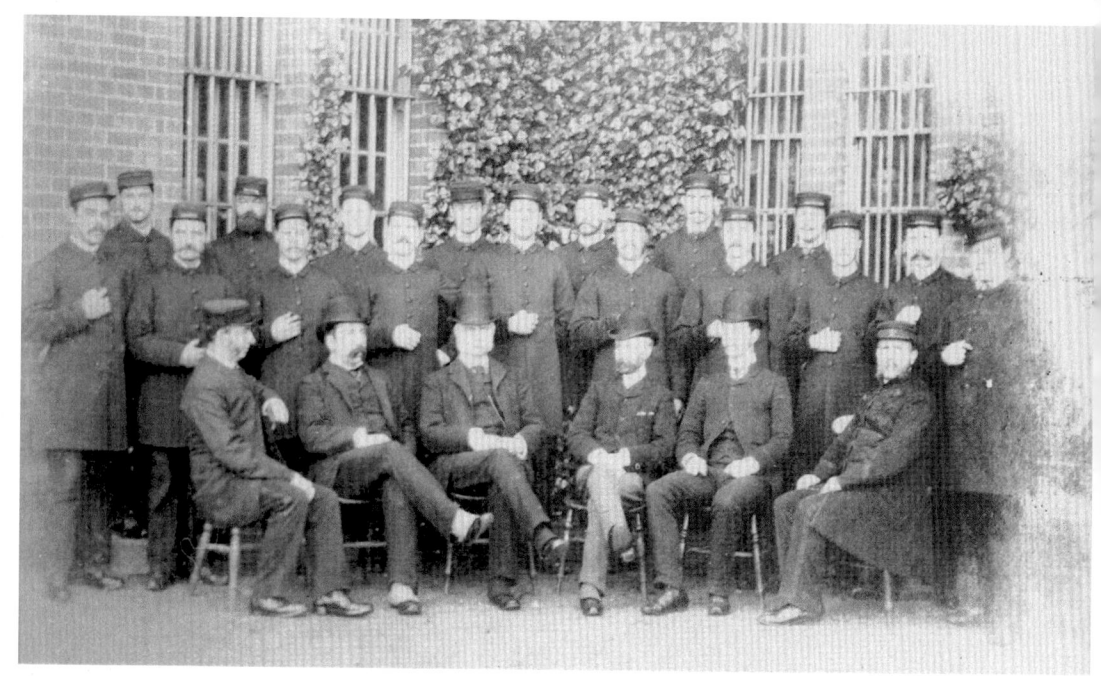

Doctors and attendants, May 1886. This less formal grouping was taken with the adjacent photograph. Here, Orange is joined only by the doctors and senior attendants. Note how the window bars blend in with the frames when viewed face on.
(*Reproduced by permission of the West London Mental Health NHS Trust/Berkshire Record Office*)

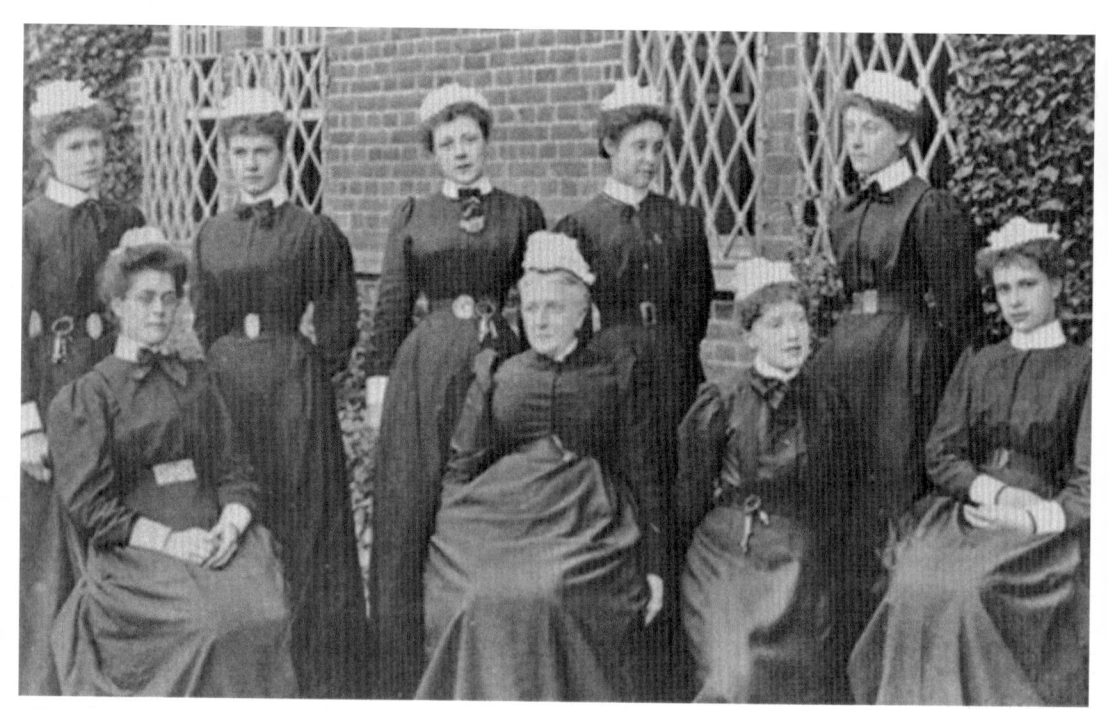

Broadmoor's female staff c.1900. This photograph shows sisters Ellen Tyman (top left) and Gertrude Tyman (seated, second from right). It was taken between 1900 and 1906, when both women were employed as attendants. In the centre is probably chief female attendant Elizabeth Morgan. She worked at Broadmoor for over 30 years, got married late in life to a senior male attendant and exceptionally was allowed to remain on the staff as a wedded woman. She retired in 1902 aged 63.
(*Privately owned, whereabouts unknown but once in the possession of Mrs Ena Pearce of Crowthorne*)

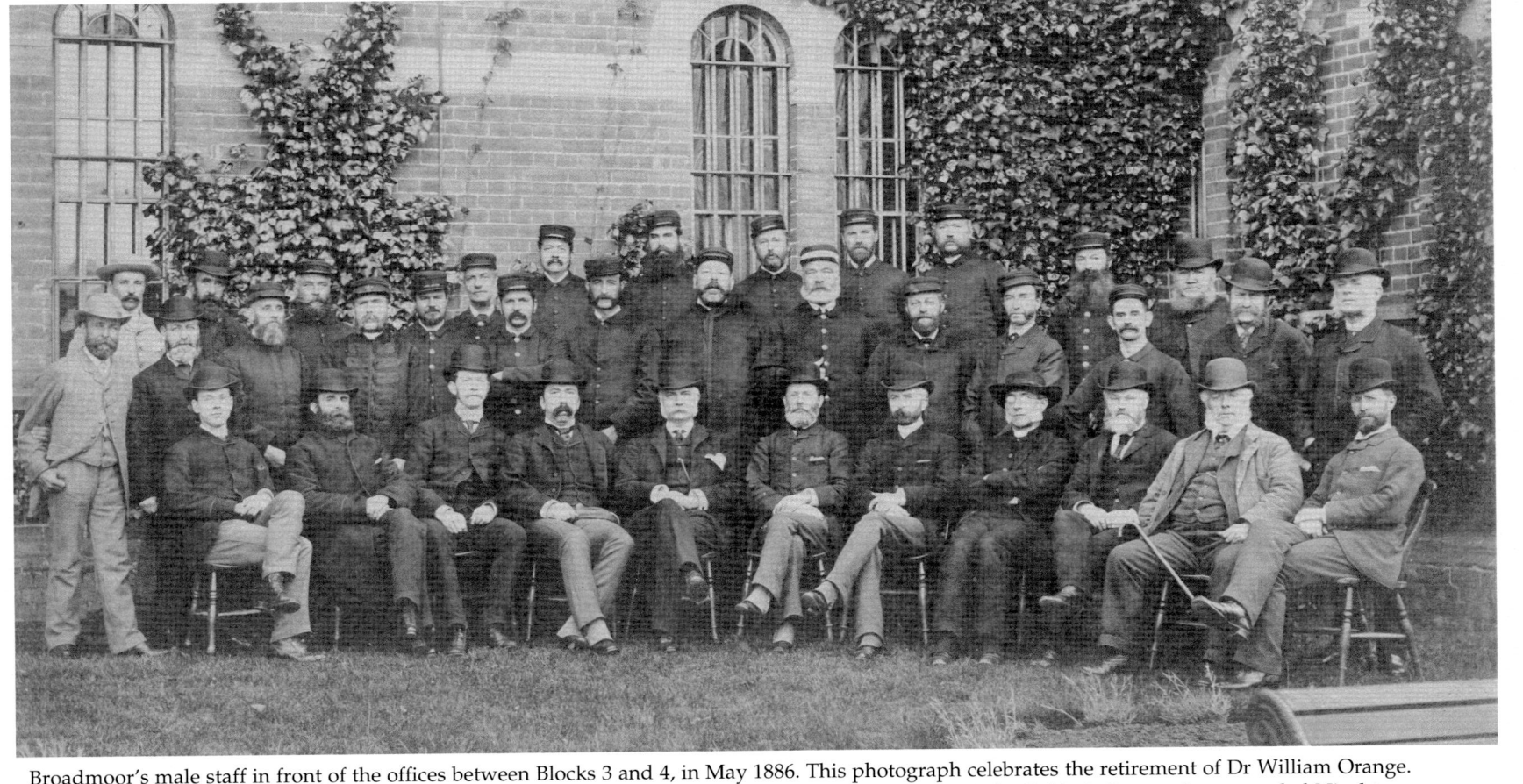

Broadmoor's male staff in front of the offices between Blocks 3 and 4, in May 1886. This photograph celebrates the retirement of Dr William Orange. Orange, wearing a top hat, is in the centre, bottom row; on his right is David Nicolson, his successor; John Baldwin Isaac, who succeeded Nicolson as Deputy Superintendent, is two away on Orange's left; junior medic Charles Paterson is to Nicolson's right; Chaplain Thomas Ashe is fourth from the right. Far right on the bottom is Charles Phelps, Asylum Steward, seated next to his son Charles, who worked in the clerks office. The other men in the front row are probably the rest of the clerks. At Isaac's right shoulder is Samuel Rawson, chief attendant, and the rest of the uniformed men in that row are probably the senior attendants. Other long-serving attendants are behind. Those in uniforms with hidden buttons would have worked in the back blocks; some wear padded jackets to protect them. (*Reproduced by permission of the West London Mental Health NHS Trust/Berkshire Record Office*)

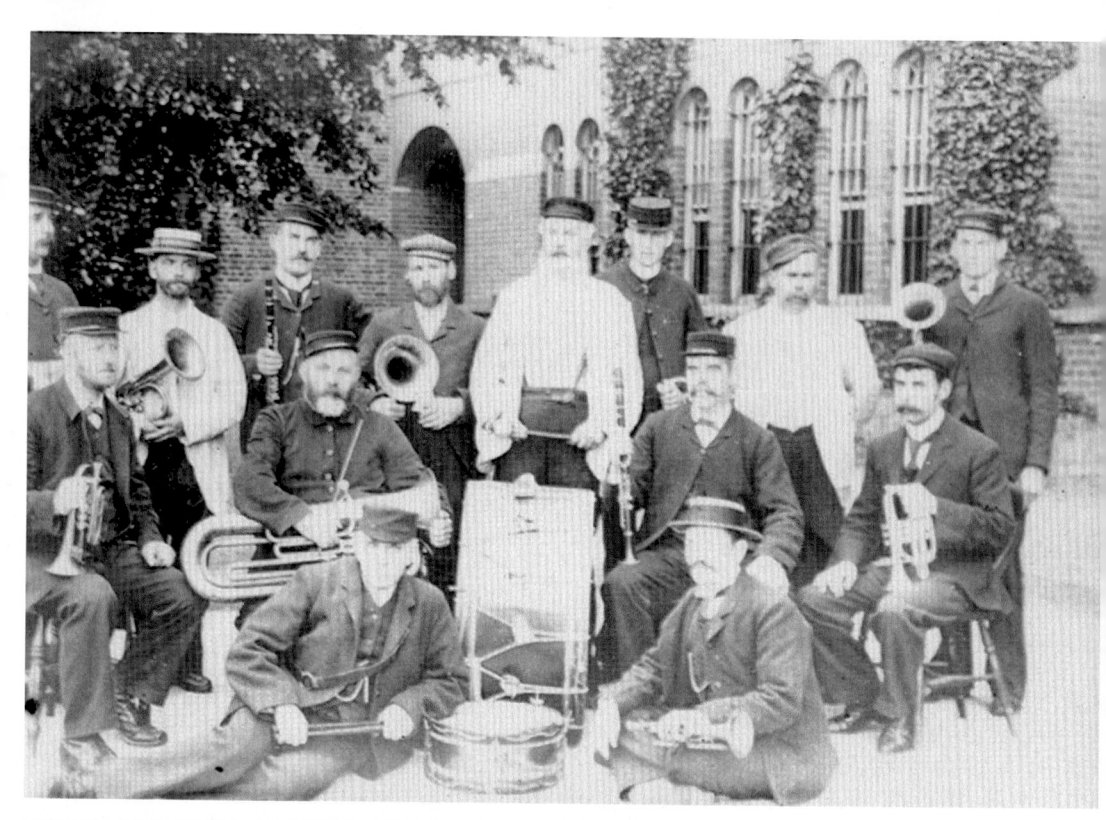

The asylum band, May 1886. The only known image of the group of staff and patients that played weekly in the asylum.
(*Reproduced by permission of the West London Mental Health NHS Trust/Berkshire Record Office*)

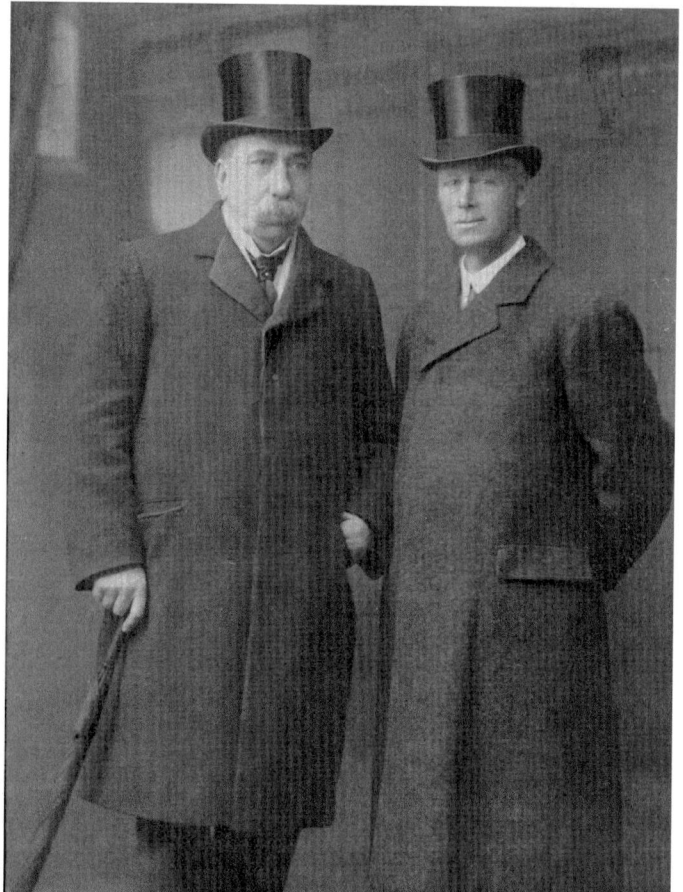

David Nicolson (*left*) and Richard Brayn (*right*), pictured in the medical superintendent's office in Broadmoor. This photograph was possibly taken on Richard Brayn's retirement in October 1910.
(*Reproduced by permission of the West London Mental Health NHS Trust/Berkshire Record Office*)

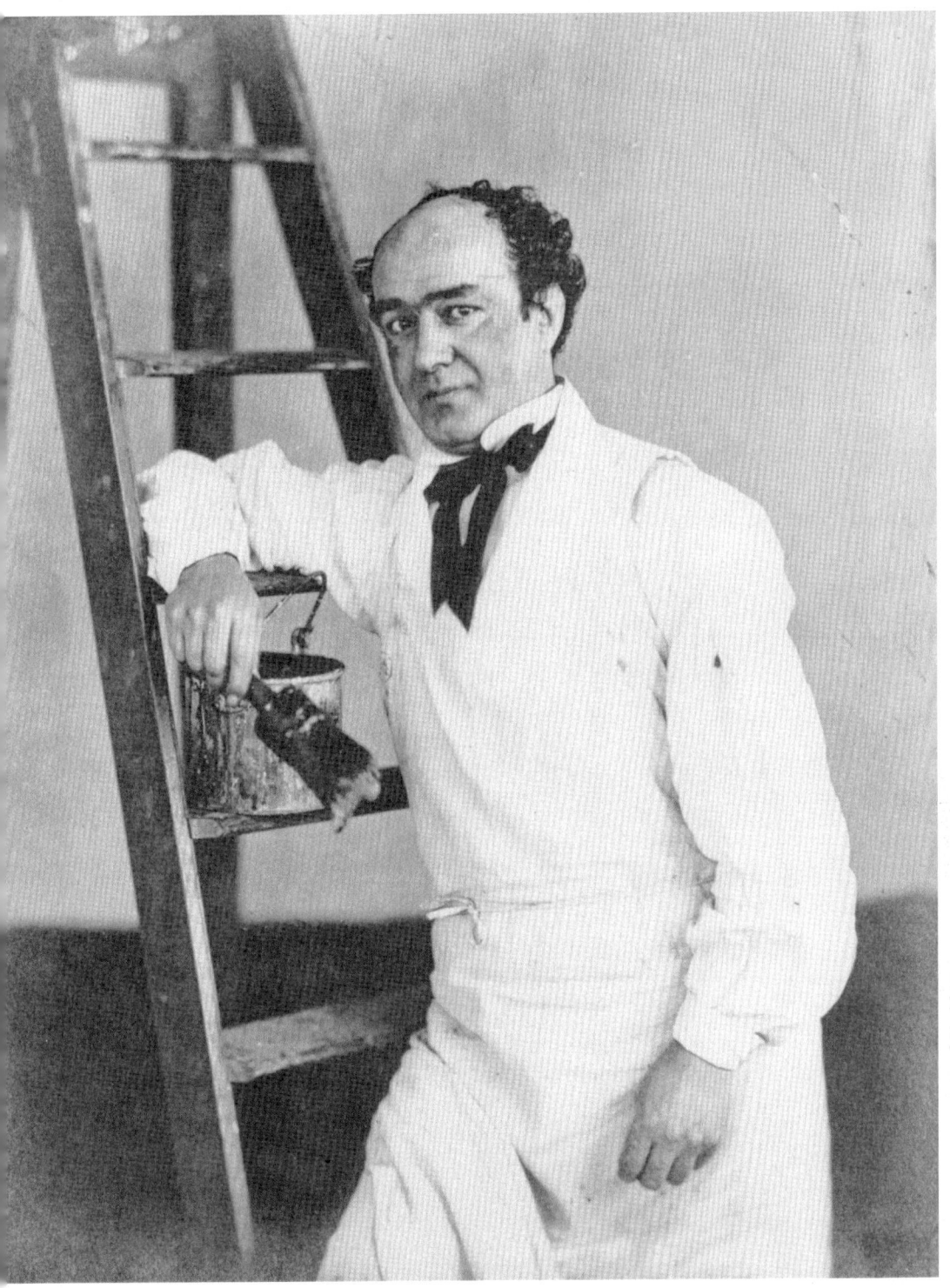

Edward Oxford in Bethlem, c.1857, photographed by Henry Hering. Oxford was no longer the callow youth who had shot at Queen Victoria. Middle-aged, he is pictured with the tools of his trade as a house painter, greeting the lens with a confident, rational gaze.
(*Reproduced by permission of The Bethlem Art and History Collections Trust*)

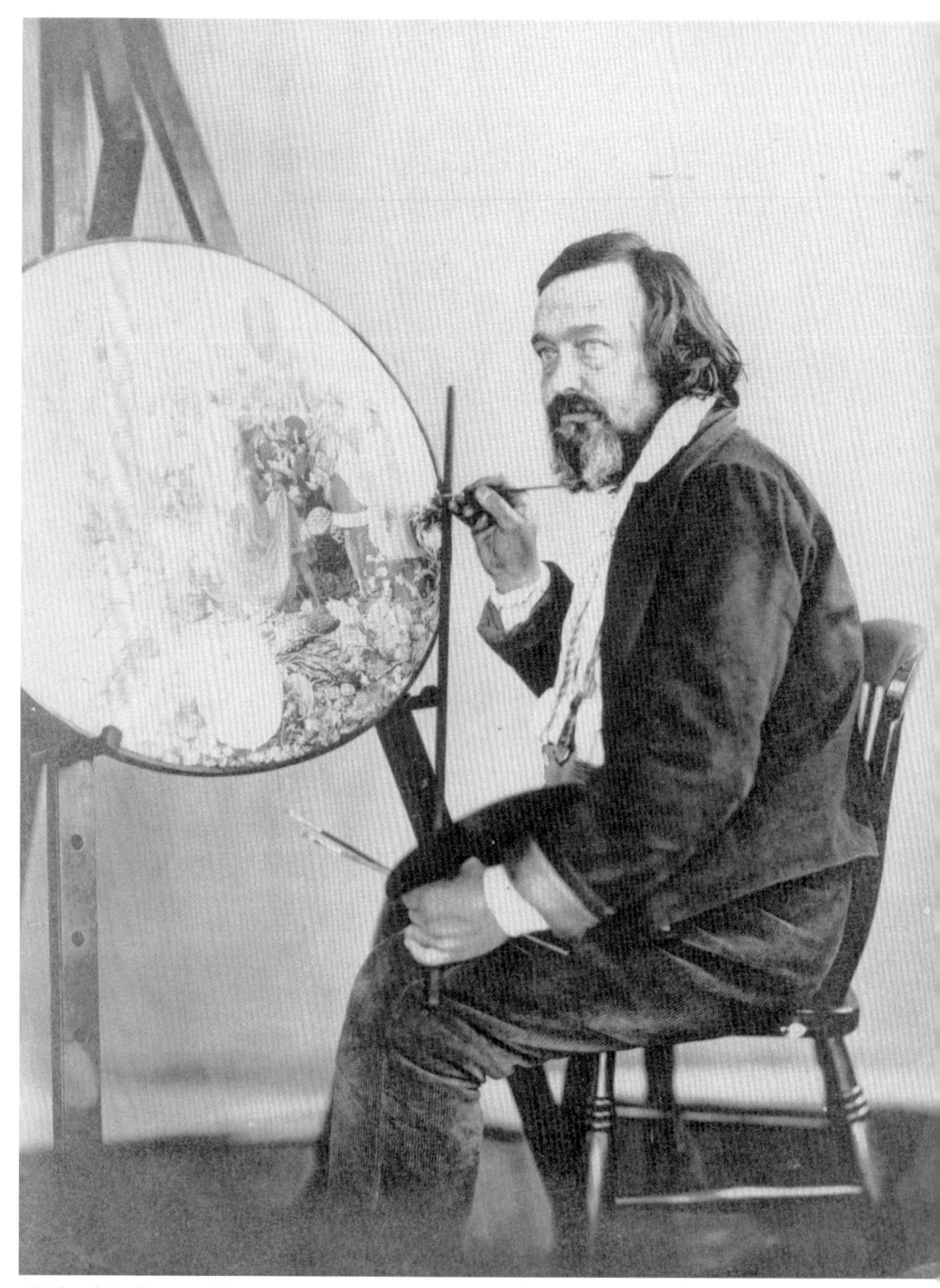

Richard Dadd in Bethlem, c.1857, photographed also by Henry Hering, while at work on 'Contradiction: Oberon and Titania', one of his finest paintings.
(Reproduced by permission of The Bethlem Art and History Collections Trust)

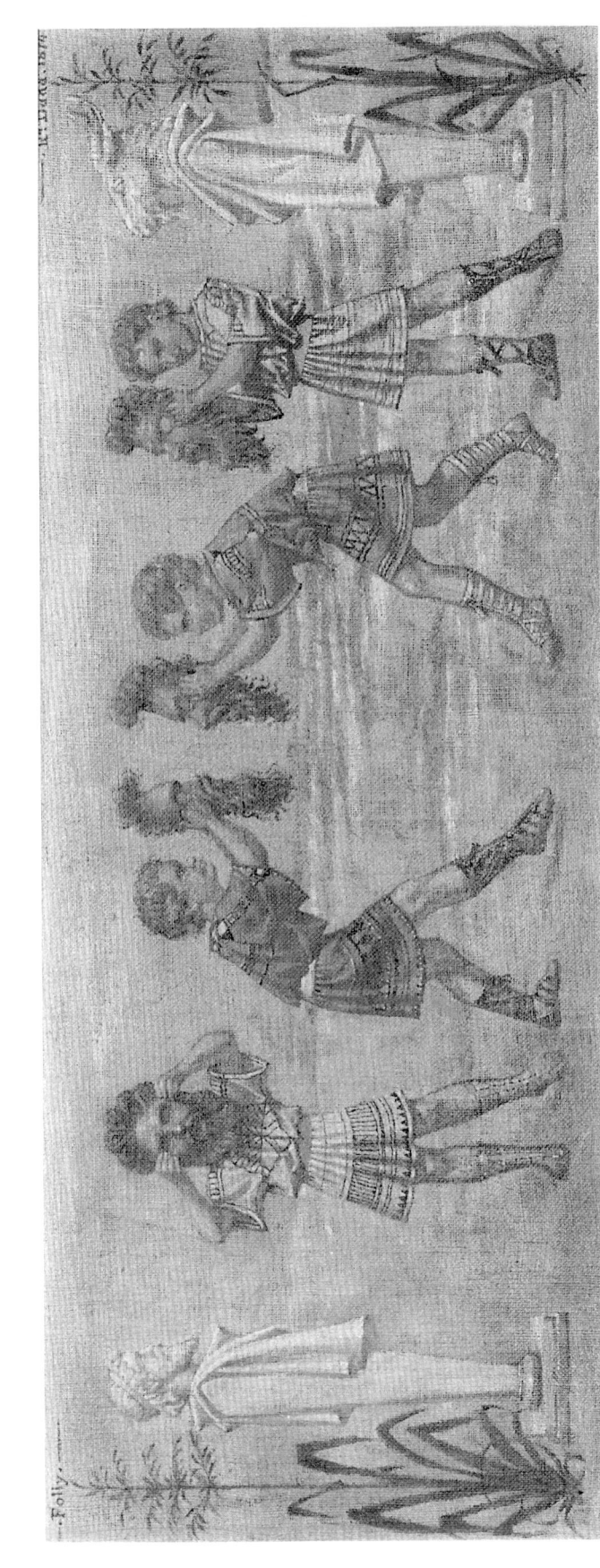

'Folly', 1874. One of six panels which Dadd painted for the front of the stage in the Broadmoor central hall. These were removed when the hall was redecorated in the early twentieth century. (*Reproduced by permission of The Bethlem Art and History Collections Trust*)

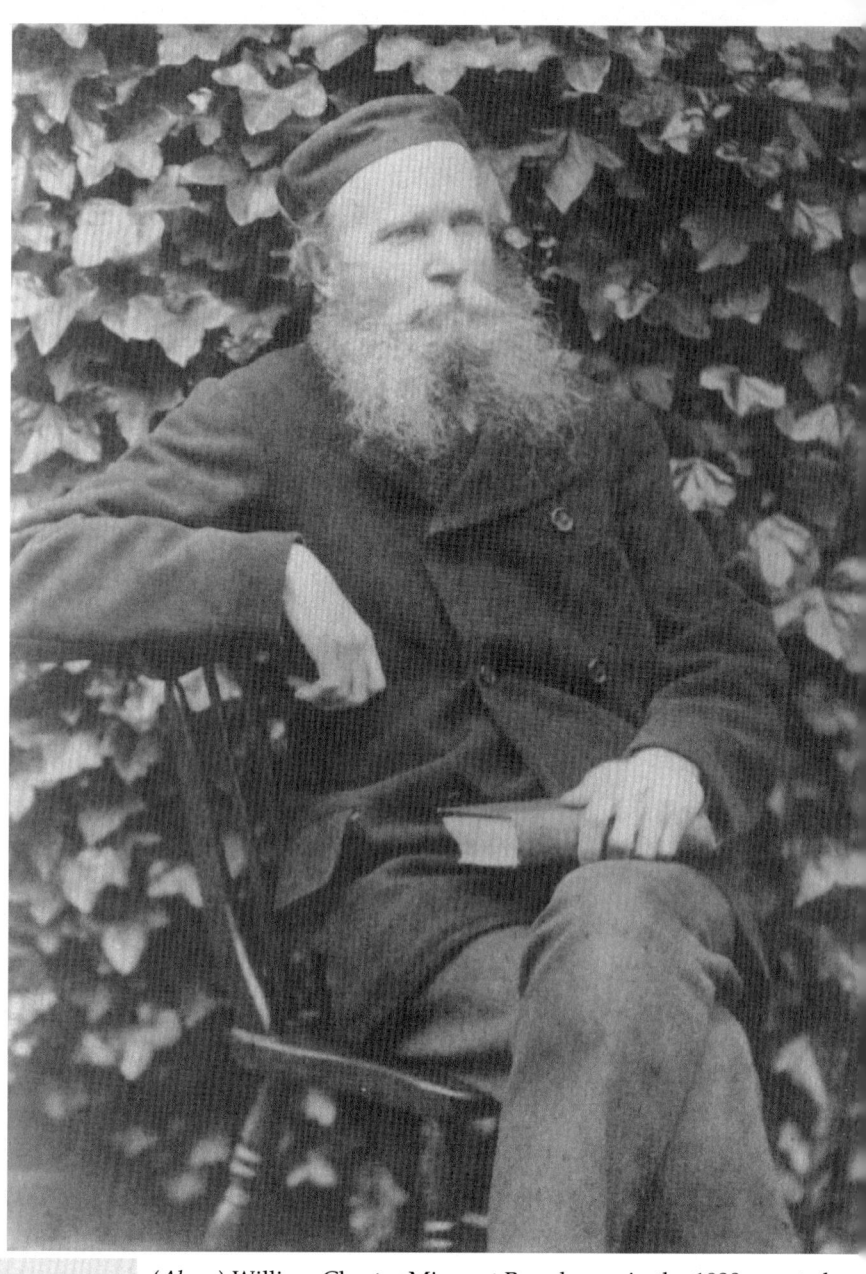

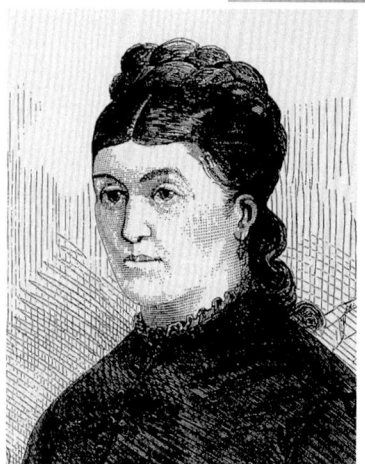

(Above) William Chester Minor at Broadmoor in the 1880s, seated close to the spot where the male staff lined up for Orange's farewell photograph. *(The Minor Family)*

(Left) Christiana Edmunds in the dock at the Old Bailey, 1872. A contemporary newspaper sketch of the 'Chocolate Cream Poisoner'.

and threw a cup of tea at him, grazing his forehead. It was all the proof that Thompson needed: there was a plot to murder him, and then throw his lifeless body overboard, where no one could find the evidence.

Thompson had a small tin biscuit box, lined with carpet, in which he stored his papers relating to the family's Carolina smallholding. Now he took that box and emptied its contents over the side of the *Peru*, so that the crew would not be able to steal his property. Then he beat the box until it was flat and placed this makeshift tin armour round his abdomen. He took two revolvers and a handful of bullets from the ship's arsenal and hid them in the kitchen. Then he turned the lights out in the galley and waited for the attack that never came.

The next morning, it was Ogilvy again who ventured onto Thompson's ground. Ogilvy wanted coffee, and proffered his pot for the cook to fill. Glancing down at the container as Thompson poured the hot liquid, Ogilvy noticed the pistol in his crewmate's hand.

"Are you allowed to carry that, cook?"

No answer. Doubtful, Ogilvy went to fetch the mate, William Orr, and when the two men returned Thompson professed innocence, claiming that it was a kitchen knife that Ogilvy had glimpsed. Yet no sooner than he made this claim, Thompson produced another pistol from his other hand and fired. The gun jammed. Sensing their chance, Ogilvy and Orr ran as Thompson squeezed the trigger. This time the weapon fired, and Ogilvy was dealt a glancing blow on his back. He turned again, faced his foe and raced back towards the galley, seeking to overpower Thompson. Now the cook reached for his other pistol and fired again, catching Ogilvy in the neck.

"You son of a bitch, you've shot me!"

There was a thundering of feet from all over the ship as crewmen arrived to corner Thompson in his lair. A siege negotiation began. Thompson was talked down from his irrational heights and a short while later was outlining to one and all the plot against his life; at the same time, Ogilvy was held down as the bullet was cut out of him. Blood poured from the wound onto the deck.

Thompson was locked up in the sail room below decks for the remaining six weeks of the voyage. Ogilvy recovered from his injuries and resumed his duties. Thompson tried to bribe Orr to throw the ship's log books overboard and forget about the whole thing. When the ship arrived in the London docks in early November, Thompson was arrested and his suit of tin was discovered on him. He maintained his story that Ogilvy and others were intending to kill him, and he was found not guilty but insane at the Old Bailey later that month.

Thompson was experiencing a complete mental breakdown. While in his Newgate Prison cell, he heard his dead uncle speak to him, and at night a vision of his three dead sisters visited him, a cluster of angels surrounded by a blazing light. He believed himself also set upon by gangs of men who beat him. These auditory and visual hallucinations were petrifying him. It was a terrifying, disorientating state to be in and he would not recover. Thompson remained fearful, and had to be repeatedly disarmed of stones that he collected in his handkerchief to aid his protection from the attendants and the other patients. He grew stout on his rations and comparative lack of manual work. His years of heavy drinking had also taken their toll on his liver. By April 1883 he was bedridden in the Broadmoor infirmary, and died that September.

Thompson's Broadmoor file ends with the thoughts of his mother, writing all the way from Charleston to ask for the return of any effects after the 'death of her only living child now lying in his cold and narrow grave'. An inventory was made: two sailor's chests, containing a Japanese wooden cabinet and a model house; a mahogany tea caddy; four oil paintings; jackets; shirts; shoes; and a cache of family letters. She would never visit her son's last resting place, so what remained of him was sent to her, while Thompson's money – five pounds and 13 shillings – was put to the use of his family back in Glasgow.

Like Thompson, sailor Joseph Peters died at Crowthorne. But before he did, he mapped out an abbreviated version of his life story in a letter dictated for Dr Orange shortly after his admission in 1877. Peters was born in Liberia, on Africa's west coast, into a great social experiment. His mother was one of a large number of freed black American slaves who had been transported to Africa through the rather mixed motives of the American Colonization Society. The society, a band of unreconstructed racists and sincere do-gooders, believed that cultural integration was unlikely to be achieved within their own country, and so the best course of action was to keep America for themselves and give the slaves the chance of a new life in another continent, far, far away. Peters's mother was a typical example of the encouraged emigrant: born and bred in Virginia, Liberia was hardly somewhere that she would have called home.

Despite the country's dubious start, and the fact that the settlers failed to integrate with the indigenous people, the US colony became a going concern. Business flourished on the short stretch of coastline that the incomers managed to command against attack. Peters's mother worked in a rice and corn processing store, and the owner of that store – 'a foreign man', is how Peters simply described him – put his mother in the family way. It was not an auspicious beginning to his life, though it could have been worse. His father did not abandon his boy, but ensured that he was found work: first in the rice store, and later as an apprentice to a carpenter friend.

Peters hated life with the carpenter, whose children were cruel to him. He was rescued by his mother and placed in school instead. Then, his father died and the rice store was commandeered by other settlers. Schooling came to an end and Peters never learned to read or write. Subsequently, his childhood took on a regular pattern of lucky break followed by ill fortune. First of all his mother met another freeman, this time from Sierra Leone, and they married. The new family unit farmed happily for a while, until the stepfather abruptly went off with another woman. Peters was reduced to selling bread and ginger beer on street corners. Through hard work and frugality they rose again, and his mother took on the rent of a shop. It was the last hurrah. For whatever reason – Peters alleged that one of the staff stole from them – that did not work out either, and soon they were destitute once more.

At the age of 16, Peters had already seen a lot of life, much of it unpleasant and challenging. Now, he chose to leave Africa and go to sea. He signed up with a trading vessel bound for London and, shortly after he arrived in port, word reached him that his mother was dead. With no remaining family, there was nothing to go back for. So he travelled all over the world on the merchant ships – to India, Africa, Australia, North and South America – and always returning to England, increasingly to Liverpool.

Yet gradually, clouds of worry began to sweep over Joseph Peters. He was locked up twice, once in Liverpool and once in London, because he had 'a little too much in my head'. Returning one time to Bristol, he had a stand-up fight with the ship's second mate, and was given one month in jail. As with Thompson, drink was undoubtedly one of Peters's demons. He spent time in a lock-up in Calcutta after he arrived drunk at the port, and endured a similar experience in Rio de Janiero. But a night in the cells in Buenos Aires convinced him that there was more to his misfortune than simply liquor. He had to be restrained when he was arrested, and during the struggle received a cut on his thumb from one of the policemen's sabres.

This cut tormented him. By the time he arrived back in Liverpool it was agony, almost certainly infected. He bought some medicine from a backstreet doctor, but it did no good. Then his ship made port at Bristol, and here he became suddenly aware of people talking about his wound behind his back. Though it might have been expected for a black man to stand out on the streets of these English cities, he had never felt remarked upon before. He was also distrustful of drugs and physicians now. The Liverpool doctor was the cause of the problem: 'He wanted five pounds, but I had only a sovereign and I said I would halve it with him, and he gave me ten shillings' worth of physic. When I took it I felt very bad and low spirited. I told him of it, and he said the five would put me alright, but I thought it wouldn't, for if a ten shilling medicine made me feel very bad, a five pound medicine would kill me outright'. With little alternative but to resume seafaring, he took another voyage to Montreal. It was a mistake. The finger bothered him more and more and on board ship he had no treatment available. The swollen abscess grew until it burst. In Canada, he decided that enough was enough and had the digit amputated.

But the phantom finger followed him. Peters noticed that now everyone was talking about him. Back in England, and then in India, he discovered to his horror that whole song books had been written about his infection. The unspoken intimation was that Joseph Peters had not been infected by a policeman's bayonet, but by a much baser kind of swordmanship encounter. Shame now accompanied Peters across the globe. His torment continued in Rangoon, in Trinidad and then back in London. Everywhere, people would nudge and wink to one another as they discussed or sang about his predicament. Increasingly he could find relief only in his cups. His drinking became heavier and heavier. After another fight he spent a few months in jail again, at Coldbath Fields in London, before embarking on his last, fateful voyage to Melbourne.

The SS *Durham* set sail for Australia in January 1877. Peters was engaged as the ship's fireman, despite the fact that he was transforming himself into his very own incendiary device. Each firework needs a spark, and Peters found one in William Barnett, the engineer on board. Laid back where Peters was highly strung, Barnett enjoyed the sport of winding up his fellow seaman before standing back to take in the show. "That's how I like to see you," Barnett said each time Peters flew into a rage.

Peters asked to be separated from Barnett when it came to sharing the watch, but was ordered to get on with his work. Eventually, he cracked. When the ship was eight days out from port on the return voyage, Peters thrust the engineer's head down onto some coals and began to pound it. Mercifully, his assault was interrupted. 'I really think I should have hurt him', he recalled, 'if a man from behind had not got hold of me'. Clapped in irons in the belly of the boat, Peters was offloaded to the magistrates and found insane.

Like all the members of the international brigade, Peters found some sort of solace in Crowthorne. He was listened to and his fears of persecution accepted for what they were. He was allowed to rest when the spirits were not bothering him, and sympathised with when they were. His errant finger was permitted to play its part in his system of values. Nor were his lack of education or sophistication held up against him. Orange used his own time to persevere with Peters's employers, Wigwam Shipowners, until they had delivered up the fireman's property and the wages he was owed. Anything that might provide a little comfort was worth pursuing and Orange had no way of knowing for how long Peters would be under his wing.

In the end, this was only a short time. Believing himself to be the victim of witchcraft, Peters ignored a growing tumour on his upper leg until it grew so large that in 1883 Orange decided intervention was required. A Reading surgeon recommended amputation up to the hip joint, and in the ensuing operation, Peters's femoral artery was severed. He died three hours after his leg was lost, and when he was buried in the asylum cemetery a few days later, aside from the staff no one came.

Peters was just another labouring man trying to make a living in difficult and lonely circumstances. The same may be said of all the patients who had come to Victorian England for business, marriage or to escape hostilities overseas. The wealth that they created would pale against Minor's family empire, for example, and judged in the crudest light their contribution to society was slight. They are linked only by the symptoms that they suffered and by the accident of birthplace instead of any deeper shared experience.

Yet one of the more intriguing aspects of the Broadmoor archive is that there are so many voices in Victorian England left unheard. The immigrant's voice may be the least heard of all. And each tale provides a sense of the diversity in what was arguably the most developed industrial society of its age. These patients also appear to have been treated just like anybody else, both within and without Broadmoor. This is not to say that Victorian England was a country free of racism, but it is very hard to find affronted newspaper reports about these patients, whose crimes more likely merited a paragraph or two lost amongst the other court reports of the day than evidence of any wider social fears.

Fear would come in time, of course, and in 1905, as the Edwardian era dawned, the first legislation was passed that aimed to restrict immigration into the British Isles, followed by many similar attempts since. It is debatable whether its terms would have prevented entry to any of the foreign patients in Victorian Broadmoor. Besides, a glance at any page of the hospital's admissions registers verifies that nationality is not of itself an accurate predictor of mental illness.

6

Christiana Edmunds: The Venus of Broadmoor

What of the women in Broadmoor? Separated on their own side of the asylum estate, they also have stories to be told. There are fewer of them in this book, reflecting the statistical imbalance of the sexes in the asylum, with roughly four men referred for every one woman. This also reflects the fact that previous investigators have found the most fascinating cases of the Victorian period to be those of men who achieved despite their illness, providing an element of atonement. Unfortunately, the same cannot be said for the most celebrated Victorian female patient, who stands out largely for negative, stereotypical, even voyeuristic reasons. Christiana Edmunds was a woman who satisfied a certain need for stories featuring sex, jealousy and vanity. She was an atypical female patient at Broadmoor, but no less newsworthy for it. The Victorian tabloids christened her 'The Chocolate Cream Poisoner'.

Christiana's background was comfortable, yet blighted. She was the eldest child of William, a local architect and Ann Christiana, a major's daughter, born in 1829 in the coastal town of Margate, Kent. The Edmunds family was sufficiently wealthy to send the children off to board at private schools and Christiana grew up in a household insulated from many of the day-to-day troubles experienced by the population at large. However, this stability did not last, for the household was also touched by mental illness. Her father went mad when Christiana was 14; sent first to a small private house in Southall and then, when the money ran out, to a much larger residence in Peckham. He died four years later. Nor was he alone. Christiana's younger brother Arthur was born with learning difficulties, and would spend the last part of his short life in the Earlswood Asylum for 'Idiots'; her sister Louisa suffered from 'hysteria' and threw herself out of a window as a young woman. The Edmunds home was unpredictable and populated by difficult behaviours. Such hereditary factors were seized on by the Victorians as strong indicators for Christiana's own diagnosis.

Her father's last years had been beset by a diminution of income, probably related to his illness as well as to a wider economic malaise, and after his death, the family was obliged to move to other quarters at Canterbury. However, they were still well off enough for Christiana's mother to maintain an independent income as a landlady and for none of her children to have to work.

Now in her late teens, Christiana grew up cosseted and cherished as a 'lady of fortune, tall, fair, handsome and extremely prepossessing in demeanour'. No doubt she was introduced to society and waited for a marriage that never came. Gradually, life moved on for the other members of the house. Her sister Mary, the only Edmunds sibling to escape the family curse, wedded a clergyman and moved to Chichester. Louisa became a governess before she died in her thirties, while Arthur's violent rages led to his absence from the age of 20 until his death six years later.

By the mid-1860s, Christiana and her mother had moved back to the seaside: to Brighton, a stone's throw from the Royal Pavilion and the beach. Life was peaceful and undemanding, with only shopping and socialising to break the routine. It was also very boring. As she passed the age of 40, Christiana remained a spinster with a little money to burn and an awful lot of time on her hands.

In the summer of 1869 she first met Dr Charles Beard. Always of a delicate constitution, Christiana needed treatment for some unspecified illness and decided to attend the physician, who lived in the townhouse opposite the Edmunds. Beard was a native of Brighton and a similar age to Christiana. What happened next is the subject of conjecture. Undoubtedly, Christiana fell head over heels, as she began to send Dr Beard love letters, at first couched in the most subtle tones. Dr Beard may not even have realised what was happening as he encouraged Christiana by replying to her. Though there was clearly no affair in a physical sense, some sort of emotional connection was made.

There was a small problem, however; Dr Beard had been married to his wife Emily for nearly ten years and had just become a father to their fourth child. Whatever the nature of this relationship with his patient, to continue it was unwise and disloyal to his wife. During the summer of 1870 the burden of deceit became too much, and Dr Beard asked Christiana to stop writing to him: 'This correspondence must cease, it is no good for either of us'.

Christiana did not stop. Aggrieved and embarrassed, she was determined to ensure that contact did not cease peremptorily. By now she had grown accustomed to calling on the Beards from time to time while on her promenades, and she used this familiarity to take an extraordinary action. One day in September 1870, Christiana visited Mrs Beard with a gift of chocolate creams. Like any polite hostess, and unaware of Christiana's business with her husband, Mrs Beard ate some of the chocolates. Afterwards she was violently sick. When Dr Beard heard of the incident, he immediately accused Christiana of poisoning his wife, although she refuted the allegation. Instead, Christiana complained that she was as much a victim as Mrs Beard, for the same chocolates had made her sick too. Perhaps Dr Beard could offer some assistance? Initially, Beard withdrew his accusation, but when Christiana still refused to tone down her devotion to him she was banished from the Beard household, after a last climactic meeting in January 1871.

If he had thought that a gentlewoman might take a gentleman at his word, then Dr Beard would soon realise that Christiana would not be eradicated from his life so easily. The love letters continued to arrive at his offices, sometimes forwarded to him from home, two or three times every week. He ignored them. This might have just become another case of a spurned lover, except that over the next few months there were further cases of people falling ill in Brighton after eating sweets and chocolates. None was newsworthy on its own, but each one featured a violent sickness, which passed quickly and without lingering harm. Stories spread by word of mouth but nobody knew the truth: that Christiana Edmunds had decided to prove her innocence of Dr Beard's accusation – by poisoning other people.

To a certain extent, this was delinquent, childish behaviour rather than anything more destructive. Only the disconnected reasoning in the motive hinted at an underlying illness. For Christiana ploughed on, aiming only at her own absolution (presumably to be followed by a fulfilling romantic consummation) as she strove to convince the doctor that she was as much a victim as anyone.

Instead things took a more serious, and unexpected turn on 12 June 1871, when a man called Charles Miller arrived on holiday in Brighton with his brother's family. Miller went to a sweet shop called J.G. Maynard, bought some chocolate creams, ate a few, and then gave one to his four year-old nephew, Sidney Barker. Miller became ill, but recovered. His small nephew died. An inquest found that the poor boy had died of strychnine poisoning. Amongst those who came forward to give evidence was Christiana, who claimed that she and her friends had also become ill after eating sweets from Maynard's store. She blamed Mr Maynard for some personal discomfort caused the previous year, when the wife of a good friend had suffered a similar bout of food poisoning. There was evidence to back this up, because tests before the inquest discovered strychnine in the chocolates sold by Maynard's. How had it got there? That question was left unanswered. A verdict of accidental death was recorded on the boy, and the shop owner John Maynard was exonerated of any intentional poisoning. He destroyed his entire stock.

The other outcome of the inquest was Christiana's vindication in Dr Beard's eyes. Or so she thought. But Christiana's constant pestering had finally driven Dr Beard to a more radical solution. He had resolved to depart for a new life in Scotland, perhaps hoping that his being out of sight would finally put him out of Christiana's twisted mind.

Christiana's carefully laid plan was in danger of being ignored. Despairing, she wrote three anonymous letters to Sidney Barker's father urging him to sue Maynard for his son's death. All the letters suggested foul play, and assured him that the 'young lady' who spoke to the inquest would be prepared to help in any further proceedings. She also continued her poisoning spree. A palpable sense of fear crept through the streets of the seaside town. Where and who would the killer strike at next? The police had no leads, and no obvious way of protecting the local population.

They decided to make a public appeal. Brighton's chief constable placed an advertisement in the local newspaper offering a reward for any information leading to the arrest of the poisoner.

That action became part of the endgame. The intrigue culminated on 10 August 1871, when six prominent local men and women, including Emily Beard, received parcels of poisoned fruits and cakes, sent by courier on a train to Brighton from Victoria Station. This time, two of Mrs Beard's servants had been invited to taste her gift, and both fell ill after eating a poisoned plum cake. The Beard household was not alone; one of their neighbours had also been poisoned, along with the editor of the local newspaper. And, once again, Christiana Edmunds had received one of the poisoner's parcels. When the police arrived to remove her own delivery, she told them that she feared for her safety: "I feel certain that you'll never find it out."

She then took up her pen and paper and wrote her last letter to Dr Beard, drawing much attention both to Mrs Beard's near miss, and to the ongoing issue of the Barker inquest. Christiana was taunting the police, and she was taunting Dr Beard. Did she want to be caught? If so, she had finally sown the seeds of her own capture. After he received that final letter Dr Beard decided to go to the police and voice his suspicion that Christiana Edmunds might have something to do with it all. He handed over the large cache of letters she had continued to write to him, even after being exiled from his presence. The fact that he had kept these letters secretly meant that they were potentially incriminating to him as well, but he must have concluded that the seriousness of the situation required him to face his own social judgement. The Brighton Police realised that Christiana's behaviour made her a potential suspect, so they decided to test out Dr Beard's theory. They wrote to her about the Barker case, and received a reply in the same hand as both the doctor's correspondence and the anonymous letters received by Barker's father.

Christiana was arrested a week after the latest batch of poisoned parcels arrived. When the police began to ask around about Miss Edmunds suddenly many small and unconnected incidents began to make sense. It did not take long to discover that she had left Brighton on Tuesday 8 August to spend two days in Margate, attending to family business. She had returned on Thursday, first catching the train to London before travelling to Brighton from Victoria. She had been placed at the scene of the crime: on the same train that had carried the poisoned post. But what exactly was the crime?

The police worked forwards from Dr Beard's letters and concluded that the motive must be sex. Christiana was demonstrably in love with Dr Beard, and had decided that her only hope lay in the removal of Mrs Beard. Christiana had taken to experimenting with strychnine in preparation for a renewed attempt to kill the obstacle to her happiness. Throughout the spring and summer of 1871 these experiments had been meted out allegedly on animals and innocent passers-by, with different dosages of poison tested and the results noted. Sidney Barker's death was the inevitable result of these experiments, and more victims would surely follow. A decision was made to prosecute, and Christiana Edmunds was charged with the attempted murder of Emily Beard.

This set the scene for her committal hearing at the Brighton Police Court one week after her arrest, on 24 August 1871. Christiana appeared decked in black, wearing a long silk dress, a lace shawl, and a veiled bonnet. Over the course of three hearings, many witnesses provided the missing pieces in the jigsaw. Dr Beard testified to the events of September 1870, when his wife had fallen sick after eating chocolates. A boy called Adam May told the court that he had run errands for Edmunds, taking forged prescriptions to druggists to obtain poisons. He was given other errands too: to purchase sweets and chocolates for her from a shop called Maynard's. A chemist called Isaac Garrett testified that he had known Edmunds as 'Mrs Wood' for four years, and that in March 1871 and on two subsequent occasions he had supplied her with strychnine. She had said she wanted to poison some local cats which were causing a nuisance. Others called to the stand placed Edmunds at the scene of even more, hitherto unrecorded, poisoning events.

Enough evidence existed to charge Christiana with a multitude of offences. All those who had received the recent poisoned gifts appeared to know the Beards or have some familiarity with the poisoning case. Perhaps she was trying to kill them all. But when the magistrates had sifted all the evidence, they noticed that at the centre of the mystery was Maynard's sweetshop. Christiana had drawn attention to Maynard's at the inquest into Sidney Barker's death, when she had provided evidence of her own poisoning. She had written to the dead boy's father urging him to prosecute the shop. She was also a known customer at the establishment, placing herself at the centre of all that had gone on in Brighton that summer. After some consideration, the direction of the prosecution changed, probably to Dr Beard's great relief. The case was no longer about his relationship with Christiana. On 7 September, Edmunds was charged with the murder of Sidney Barker, and on this new charge she would stand indicted.

The story now suggested by the prosecution was that after Christiana's failed attempt to poison Emily Beard, her subsequent activities had aimed to blame Maynard's for the whole affair and deflect attention from herself. By creating another monster she could reassure Charles Beard of her innocence. In truth no one was really sure what she had hoped to achieve, whether to continue an affair or merely create mischief. Whatever her real intentions, it was all sensational stuff and the notion of Christiana's unrequited love driving her to murder was eagerly consumed by the press.

Christiana captured the imagination of the media in a way that many Broadmoor patients did not. Column after column was dedicated to her, and though at first the case was scheduled to be heard at the Lewes Assizes, close to Brighton, it was felt impossible to find a jury who would not be prejudiced by what they had read in the newspapers. Instead, Christiana was taken by train to Newgate Prison in London, and her case was scheduled for the Old Bailey on the 15 and 16 January 1872.

Christiana's reputation preceeded her, and the circumstances of the case had set tongues wagging all over the metropolis. When the day arrived for her trial to begin, it was not surprising to find the courtroom full of journalists and other onlookers who had braved the bitter winter weather. Their heroine did not disappoint, appearing once more resplendent in black, this time velvet with a fur trim. She was bareheaded, as a penitent might be, and though her age was stated to be 35, her audience could see that she might actually be considerably older. Her thick black hair was parted centrally and plaited down the back of her head. *The Times* reporter was rather uncomplimentary, suggesting that she had a 'long and cruel' chin, and that her lower jaw was 'massive, and animal in its development'. Despite that, he was prepared to concede that 'the profile is irregular, but not unpleasing', and that there was 'considerable character in its upper features'. Her lips occasionally pressed together in a look of 'comeliness' that turned to 'absolute grimness' when the facts of the case were discussed. Thus was a portrait painted of a woman who thought herself more than she was; an amatory, predatory woman who used sex as a weapon. This caricature has stayed with her ever since.

That Christiana was manipulative cannot be denied. It seems certain that she would have viewed her court appearance as a performance. As she was watched by all and sundry, she took copious notes of proceedings, straining to pay attention to the detail, her dark eyes flashing occasionally as she fixed a witness with a stare, before she dipped her pen into the inkwell. Unusually, she sat in the dock, like a queen on a throne rather than a prisoner on trial.

The evidence of poisons and puddings and love gone bad uncovered at the earlier committal hearings was now repeated. More witnesses had come forward to say that Christiana had sent boys to buy sweets for her from Maynard's shop. Her *modus operandi* was finally unveiled: shortly after purchasing the sweets she would return some of them, claiming that the wrong ones had been purchased. These sweets, injected with strychnine, would then be returned to their jar for resale. Other witnesses had also seen her leave bags of sweets lying around in shops and public places. She had clearly not targeted all of her victims but left their misfortune to greed and chance.

Christiana's barrister set up the defence of insanity. Several well-known authorities testified on her behalf. Dr William Wood of Bethlem argued that she satisfied the principal MacNaughten Rule: she could not distinguish right from wrong. Dr Henry Maudsley, the famous psychologist, stated that she belonged to the 'morally defective' group of lunatics, emotionally disabled people who could not understand the harm they caused or were ambivalent to it. Then Christiana's mother took the stand to deliver the long tale of family madness, which had eventually trapped her eldest daughter. This was the only time Christiana reacted to proceedings. She cried out: "This is more than I can bear", as her mother laid open the family secrets.

In the end, it was an insanity defence which could provide no evidence of irrational delusions or beliefs. This was seized upon by the prosecution and taken up further by Lord Martin, the judge. For the first time in her life, Christiana's social standing counted against her. 'A poor person is seldom inflicted by insanity,' observed Martin, 'while it is common to raise a defence of that kind when people of means are charged with the commission of crime.' Did Christiana really not know right from wrong, or was she just oblivious to it? When the jury was asked to consider their verdict, they took an hour before they found Christiana Edmunds guilty of murder. They did not recommend mercy.

The defendant remained in the dock to hear her fate. Neatly dressed, she had added a pair of black gloves to her courtroom attire, and re-arranged her hair in a 'coquettish' manner. Before sentence was passed she was asked whether she had anything to say. She replied that she wished to be tried on the original charge of attempting to murder Emily Beard too, so that she might describe the nature of her relationship with Dr Beard: "It is owing to the treatment I received in going to him that I have been brought into this dreadful business. I wish the jury had known the intimacy, his affection for me, and the way I have been treated." If she was to go down, she surmised, then he would go down beside her. It was, of course, too late for that.

As Martin donned the black cap, Christiana faced the gallows alone. Her immediate response was fittingly dramatic: she walked slowly and deliberately up to the bar, raised her dampening eyes towards the judge and claimed that she was pregnant. It was the only card left for her to play: legal tradition meant that a pregnant woman could not be hanged until after she had given birth. Another great murmur erupted around the court. It was perfect theatre. Immediately, in line with the tradition, the court officials began to cry out for women of a certain age to make themselves known. A jury of matrons was duly gathered from the spectators in the room, and retired together with the Newgate doctor to examine Christiana in an anteroom. The courtroom emptied. Everyone waited. An hour later, Christiana was back in the dock. Asked for their verdict, the new female jury declared that Christiana was not pregnant. The law would take its course.

She returned to Lewes Prison to suffer the extreme penalty of the English legal system. But the medical evidence presented at her trial had not gone unnoticed, and incredibly, there was also some popular local sentiment towards sparing Christiana's life. On 23 January 1872, Dr Orange and Sir William Gull from Guy's Hospital visited her in prison at the Home Office's request. They conducted a long interview with her and formed conclusions broadly in agreement with the medical men who had attended her trial. Their final report to the Home Secretary summarised Christiana's case:

'This woman appears to have had a tranquil, easy and indifferent childhood and womanhood up to a period of about three years ago ... The acts were the fruit of a weak and disordered intellect with confused and perverted feelings of a most marked insane character ... The crime of murder she seems incapable of realising as having been committed by her though she fully admits the purchasing and distributing the poisons as set forth in the several counts against her. On the contrary she even justifies her conduct.'

They declared her to be insane and, after some consideration, the Home Secretary Henry Bruce respited her sentence.

In fact, he did rather more than that, for he effectively overturned the verdict of the jury. It was not uncommon to have the death sentence commuted to life imprisonment, and various other Broadmoor murderers had been transferred to the asylum with such a tariff. Their guilt, however, remained. Christiana's guilt was removed entirely, her absolution granted, contrary to the result in the courtroom. She was now considered not guilty but insane, and given the indefinite pleasure sentence. *The Times* bemoaned this unsatisfactory situation in a leader piece on 25 January, even if it did grudgingly agree that the outcome had been the right one. The paper also questioned the wisdom of politicians in permitting a jury to give 'a solemn verdict which they know will be afterwards reversed'.

Politically, the decision was unpopular everywhere. Back in Brighton, the local ratepayers soon realised that the Home Secretary had saddled them with Christiana's upkeep, as the legal place of settlement was obliged to make a contribution to a lunatic held elsewhere. To others it may have seemed fitting that such an exceptional case had resulted in such an exceptional outcome. However, the irony that her verdict could be legally correct yet medically unsound was probably of secondary importance to Christiana, after the extra attention it had garnered for her. Gull and Orange had given her back her life, and she waited eagerly for the train to take her up to Broadmoor, where she arrived on 5 July 1872.

On her admission to the asylum, Christiana was 43 years old and fighting it. She was wearing make-up on her rouged cheeks, a wig ('a large amount of false hair', is how it was described in her notes) and had false teeth. 'She is very vain', wrote Orange as he began his acquaintance with Christiana's affectations. The surgeon at Lewes Prison who signed her transfer form made his own opinions of her clear. He was unimpressed with the diagnosis of insanity, writing that after ten months of supervision he could not be satisfied either that Christiana was insane, or that she was not responsible for her actions. He did, however, say that she was of a delicate constitution and prone to hysteria.

Orange was nevertheless convinced that he had made the correct diagnosis. Christiana's behaviour in his charge did not conform to social norms. When her surviving uncle died shortly after her admission, she appeared to be completely unmoved by the loss. She was also deceitful. As soon as she was transferred, she immediately began to try to have clothes or beauty aids smuggled in to the asylum. Her younger sister Mary was complicit in this. One letter from Christiana asked for clothing; another talked about ways to apply make-up while in the asylum. Mary sent along whatever she could muster and when she visited, brought more. Orange attempted to reason with Mary, insisting that Christiana was able to partake of any comfort that she required and that it could be procured for her on the usual system of private patient accounts.

It was to no avail. Christiana kept encouraging Mary to send gifts, much to the increasing irritation of the matron of Broadmoor's female wing. Inside every parcel that came to Christiana was some sort of contraband, often hidden within another item. Each one needed time and attention to unpick and search. It was as if there was an attention-seeking conspiracy on the part of the Edmunds women, and it was more than the matron could bear. The final straw was a cushion stuffed with false hair, which arrived during the summer of 1874. The matron complained to Orange that Christiana had been amassing and hoarding hair in her room, presumably to make into new wigs, and that the room was now fit to burst with it. She pleaded that no further gifts should be allowed. Orange was initially reluctant to interfere with behaviour he saw as self-indulgent but largely harmless and possibly of occupational value. The matron, however, put her foot down. She had to clear up the hair, after all.

Also in 1874, Broadmoor intercepted clandestine correspondence sent to the chaplain at Lewes Prison, with whom Christiana had obviously attempted to strike up a bond during her time in custody. There was no problem with her writing to the chaplain (unless he objected), but Orange noted wearily that Christiana's decision to do so through some sort of secret route was 'in conformity with her state of mind to prefer mystery and concealment'. It was all just a game to Christiana. Perhaps the chaplain was intended to become a Dr Beard substitute. Still, the webs of intrigue continued. In 1875 her room was twice searched and various concealed articles were recovered and removed. Orange wrote on one of these occasions, 'she deceives for the pure love of deception'.

Christiana was certainly a patient who required micro-management. She was also a bundle of contradictions. Generally quiet and biddable, she joined the ranks of the more trusted patients in the original female block. She had access to the terrace and the gardens, and probably revelled in causing trouble while playing croquet and other games with her fellow patients. For the other side of her manipulative activities was a disruptive nature. A note of 1876 recorded that 'her delight and amusement seem to be in practising the art of ingeniously tormenting several of the more irritable patients, so that she could always complain of their language to her whilst it was difficult to bring any overt act home to herself'. If you did not pay attention to Christiana, then she would kick up some sort of rumpus to ensure that you did.

This vanity and narcissism also manifested itself in her appearance. When her mother visited, she would omit her make-up and

Christiana Edmunds: The Venus of Broadmoor

try to look as desperate as possible. If one of the male doctors was visiting the wards, her object was exactly the opposite. Christiana's make-up appears often in her notes. She was evidently perceived by the male doctors as Broadmoor's painted lady, and as a creature motivated by desire. They were the only men in regular contact with her, and she appears to have been determined to maximise their romantic inclinations. A note made in 1877 by Dr Nicolson, as Christiana approached the age of 50, related her daily life as one of embroidery and etching. But he also maintained that she 'affects a youthful appearance' and that 'her manner and expression evidently lies towards sexual and amatory ideas'. It seems certain that at the annual Christmas dance for female patients, Christiana was as bedecked and garlanded as the walls of the central hall. No doctor or male attendant would have escaped a dance with her.

Her life at Broadmoor continued in this vein for another 30 years. She presented no danger to any staff or patients and showed no obvious signs of insanity. As age slowed her, she also became a little less disruptive. She made herself up, she demanded acknowledgement, and she continued to show no remorse for her crimes, but otherwise she sewed and painted; she was quiet and well-behaved. Her remaining family died and her contact with the outside world ended. Far away from Crowthorne Dr Beard, who had moved up to Southport in the aftermath of the poisoning scandal, returned home to Brighton with Emily. Christiana had been forgotten.

Perhaps if she had been one of the Broadmoor women who had acted while suffering from post-natal depression or some other recognised Victorian female illness, she might have been discharged. But there was no clamour for that, nor any regular petitions to the Home Office from her or others, no letters in the newspapers or campaigning friends to ask questions on her behalf. Orange even noted casually in 1884 that he did not actually have any paperwork authorising her detention, because the Treasury Solicitor had lost it all. He was disinclined to trouble anyone to recreate it. Nicolson wrote in 1892 that he had seen no change in Christiana during the 15 years that he had known her, and was not expecting to see any. It never seems to have crossed anyone's mind that she might rejoin society.

Now that Christiana was in her seventies, gradually her health weakened. In 1900, she was bedridden for a while with flu. By 1901 her sight was fading badly, and she could barely see out of her right eye. Her mobility decreased, and in the winter of 1906 she could hardly stand up or walk. As she entered the last year of her life, a final Christmas ball approached. Laid up in the infirmary, the ramifications of this played on Christiana's fading mind. A rather sad snippet of conversation between her and another patient was recorded by the medical staff:

Edmunds:	How am I looking?
A:	Fairly well.
Edmunds:	Are my eyebrows alright?
A:	Yes.
Edmunds:	I think I am improving. I hope I shall be better in a fortnight. If so, I shall astonish them; I shall get up and dance – I was a Venus before and I shall be a Venus again!

She died nine months later on 19 September 1907, aged 78. The cause of death was given as senile decay. Though that was the end of her physical life, the curious nature of Christiana's case had a lasting effect on many of the professionals around her. She appeared in many legal and medical textbooks, and was also apparently the inspiration for the career of the great English barrister Sir Edward Marshall Hall. Aged 13, Marshall Hall had been present at the Brighton Police Court when Christiana made her first appearance and was captivated by the woman in black before him.

Her story has also lent itself to dramatisation. She was the subject of an ITV Saturday Night Theatre film as part of its *Wicked Women* season in 1970, where Anna Massey starred as Christiana. She was also the star of *The Great Chocolate Murders* on Radio 4 in 2006, and recently became part of Steve Hennessy's series of Broadmoor plays. In Brighton, Christiana and the other characters in her story are still well-known and she has become a local legend. An enduring sense of mystery ripples through the tale, for the story still feels incomplete. Christiana remains a character whose disordered personality often seems within grasp but then disappears beyond reach. Because she never denied her actions, nor offered up an explanation of what she was trying to achieve, she has left her followers dangling.

Christiana would be delighted with this outcome. She thrived on the publicity and intrigue that her criminal actions generated, along with the thrill of the secrets that attached themselves to her affair. Perhaps her motive was no more than to enjoy all these undercover experiences, to feel life fully without caring about the consequences for others. In that sense, this unusual woman cannot be neatly reduced to the stereotype of a frustrated spinster whose desires eventually destroyed her. If so, she might be expected to have held a lasting love for Dr Beard. No evidence exists for that: she does not appear to have ever tried to correspond with him after August 1871, nor mentioned him once at Broadmoor. She simply moved onto other fun and games.

It may be that her indifference was a reaction to her surroundings. Shut away for years, she made do with whatever opportunities for personal projection and subterfuge came her way, otherwise disengaged from everything around her. As a result, there is still not enough of her in the records to show the true Christiana, and she has left us with only shards of the mirror that once contained her true reflection. The search to discover the Venus of Broadmoor continues.

7

Broadmoor Babies

When Christiana Edmunds was plunged into the female blocks at Broadmoor, she found a group of women suffering from a rather different set of symptoms to her own. These symptoms were similar to those experienced by the majority of the men, but the women were not judged in the same way. The average Victorian alienist was prepared to accept some crucial feminine periods of life – puberty, childbirth, menopause – as being potential causes of insanity, even if they did not yet understand how such events might become catalysts for sickness. Women were distinct from men, that much was clear.

Whatever the cause, the criminal outcome of a female case of insanity usually fell into two categories: habitual thieving, alcoholism or other compulsive behaviours; or murderous assaults. The former sent the greater bulk of the women convict patients to Broadmoor, and the latter the greater bulk of the pleasure women. Amongst the murderers or would-be assassins it was most unusual to find a case of stranger killing. The celebrated Miss Edmunds sat virtually alone. Generally, the victims had been their closest friends or relatives, those with whom they shared a roof, a bed or an even stronger bond.

These women dominated their smaller side of the asylum. The result was a curiously typical profile of a Broadmoor female on admission. Unlike the male wing, where the new patients ranged from children and adolescents to pensioners, in the female quarters the vast majority were of childbearing age. Any older women on the ward had simply been there a long time, and the casual observer could probably have placed a bet on how many years each one had been in Crowthorne. This is where Broadmoor differed from the city and county asylums that sprang up during the nineteenth century. In many ways, its population was a carbon copy of the national one. Only the indefinite 'pleasure' women sent by the courts and the Home Office could not be said to be truly representative.

This was partly true also of their backgrounds. Many of the patients were working women and of those who were married, their husbands were often employed in less remunerative occupations. There were not the same middle and upper class fraternities as there were on the male side of Broadmoor. Christiana would have felt far superior to many of her cohort and perhaps this explains her use of the other patients for amusement. Her rare status was evidence of the theory that middle class Victorian women, when tempted by a lunatic impulse, were prevented from its operation by male relatives or servants. If they were sent anywhere, it would be to a private house for treatment, but equally they might be nursed at home.

Of the women in more straitened circumstances who were admitted to Broadmoor, by far the greater proportion of them were the rare, but regular, Victorian mothers who attacked their own children. So many entries in the asylum's admissions register are followed by the note 'murder of her child' that after a while the phrase almost ceases to have meaning. Victorian juries were very ready to accept a defence of insanity to a crime of infanticide.

But some of these women would also give life after arriving at Broadmoor. The asylum was no different to any other institution housing women of childbearing age. Like a workhouse, prison or charitable refuge, it admitted women according to set criteria, regardless of whether or not they were pregnant. The same was true of local asylums, but although the average local asylum would have admitted plenty of patients who had just experienced childbirth, they very rarely received women who went on to have their babies within the institution. Generally, the local asylums were seen as best avoided during pregnancy. Broadmoor, of course, could not exercise the same choice, bound as it was by judicial process, and so neither could its patients. Consequently, these events were dealt with as just another part of ward life, entirely in keeping with the ethos of this self-contained community.

This was possible because of the great divide within the asylum. The female side operated very much as an independent unit. The initial women's block and its later companion were separated from the male side to the west by a high dividing wall. There was a dedicated body of staff of around 20 female attendants to nurse the residents of these blocks, with a female operational head, although she was expected to defer to the male medical staff. There might have been a queen on the throne, but Victorian England remained patriarchal, and so too did the medical staff at Broadmoor. They frequented their offices on the men's side and made ward visits to the female patients when they wished. In their charge, notionally at least, were around 100 lunatic women.

For most of the time, the male and female patients were barely aware of each other's existence. Work and entertainment were separate. The result was a parallel, segregated life on either side of Broadmoor. The women sewed and looked after the laundry, they promenaded along their terrace or the wider grounds; they read in the day room and conversed; or, if they were in the female back block, they were minded and managed in much the same way as their aggressive counterparts in the other half of the site. Even at recreational events, such as the flower show or annual ball, the women were permitted to mix only with male staff, and not male patients. The logic in creating a rather artificial situation – a world bereft of men or women – was that it provided what was considered a safe environment for initial recovery, and one where the appropriate refuge could be given to help a patient progress. It was into this single-sex regime that all the women were transported, including those who arrived pregnant.

The first patient to give birth in the asylum was Catherine Dawson, on 26 December 1866, three and half years after Broadmoor opened. At one o'clock in the morning, surrounded by attendants, in the pale glow of gaslight she was delivered of a baby boy in the female infirmary ward. Her labour lasted only half an hour.

Catherine was in many ways a typical Broadmoor female patient of the murderous class. When she was younger, her family had moved from rural Ireland to the industrial north-west of England. Married at 17, now she was 31 years old and already a mother as well as a working class housewife. Her husband Henry was on his second marriage and the itinerant family followed his work wherever it took them. Henry's trade was looking after the coal fires that powered cranes and other stationary engines, while Catherine worked from home as a dressmaker.

There had been signs of impending trouble a few years before she arrived in Crowthorne. In 1862, while the family was living in Manchester, Henry had become so worried about his wife's propensity for violent outbursts that Catherine had been packed off to the workhouse at Ashton-under-Lyne for ten days of observation. When she returned home, he sent Catherine and their three daughters, Mary, Matilda and Harriet, off to her father in Liverpool so that she could be watched.

Henry followed soon after and took a job in the Liverpool docks, while the Dawsons rented two rooms in a shared house in Toxteth Park. This basic, hand-to-mouth existence lasted for six months. On 27 October 1864, neighbours heard a piercing scream emanate from the Dawsons' rooms, where Catherine had cut the throat of her middle child, 22-month-old Matilda, before attempting to cut her own. She was found beside the hearth with four-year-old Mary pinned between her mother's thighs, cowering as a knife was held above her. Catherine was pushed to the ground and the older child rescued. Baby Harriet was found unharmed beneath the blankets in the bedroom. Catherine was not considered fit enough to plead in her defence.

Although Broadmoor had opened 18 months previously, Catherine was transferred initially to Rainhill Asylum in Liverpool. It was rare for a pleasure patient to be accommodated outside Broadmoor or its predecessor hospitals, and Catherine must have been considered manageable in a local refuge instead. This turned out to be a misjudgement, for after 15 months at Rainhill, Catherine managed to escape. She was eventually discovered back with Henry and the remaining girls, though because the family had moved it took a month to track them down. After her return to Rainhill it was decided to move her to more secure accommodation, and she was presented at the Broadmoor gate on 15 May 1866.

On arrival in Crowthorne she was immediately sick in the waiting room, and after her details were taken she was confined to bed in the female infirmary, dosed with beef tea and effervescing salts. The sickness was initially ascribed to a phial of morphine administered to keep her calm during the long train journey south. But when the sickness did not subside the Broadmoor doctors concluded the true cause. During her month at large she had resumed her marital obligations, and become pregnant.

Unfortunately Catherine was aggressive, quarrelsome and paranoid, imagining that tricks were being played on her and determined to avenge them. When her morning sickness eventually passed she was moved to the ward for more disturbed patients and occupied herself with needlework and suspicion until she gave birth. The act of nativity itself was almost entirely unremarkable: in fact, the only statement Catherine made at the time of birth was that there was 'a nasty smell in the room'. Her baby boy was immediately removed from her after the birth and handed over to one of the attendants, who reared him on cow's milk. As Catherine was in no fit mental state to name her child, and the boy had been born on Boxing Day, the Broadmoor chaplain christened him after the Feast of St Stephen.

Catherine did not ask to see her child until a week after the birth, and not until two months had passed was she finally allowed to do so. Their first, and almost certainly only, meeting was not a success. Catherine placed little Stephen on his legs and let him go, waiting for him to walk. After the baby fell she spoke to him as if he could respond. Perhaps she was seeing an older girl in front of her, one who might have been playing in a back yard in Liverpool. There was clearly little point in trying to bond and when the boy was taken away from her again, this time it was for good.

Dr John Meyer, Broadmoor's first medical superintendent, had begun to plan arrangements for the baby's life away from his mother. His plan was to ask either Catherine's local workhouse, or her husband Henry to take Stephen into their care. He wrote to both. Henry Dawson replied clearly and convincingly that he was reluctant to accept his newborn son on the grounds of poverty. Now lodging in Birkenhead, he was out all day working by the Mersey, leaving the surviving girls with neighbours, and returning only at night with the money to feed them. But as one door closed, another remained open. The Chorley Union Workhouse had a series of questions for Meyer as to their liability for upkeep of a lunatic's child, particularly as Catherine's settlement there had been fleeting, but at no point did they refuse to offer their support. After further correspondence, the officers of the workhouse were persuaded to take on the boy. A date for his removal was fixed, and Stephen was collected from Broadmoor on 25 February 1867 and taken back to Lancashire.

The Dawson family was now split across three locations. Stephen went to the workhouse and an uncertain future. Henry and the girls remained in Birkenhead. Catherine stayed in Broadmoor, her moods swinging between excitement and depression. When she was better, she kept in contact with her husband, reading his letters and writing replies. But as well as her mental illness, she was often in poor physical health and unable either to write or work at her sewing. She would lay in bed, exhausted, with her hands and wrists scarred from time spent breaking windows in the female block. During one such period, in 1871, Henry worried that the long silence from his wife meant that she was dead. He wrote to the Broadmoor authorities asking whether his wife was still living. Shortly after it was confirmed that she was, he visited her.

It was to be their last meeting. Though Catherine Dawson was slowly failing it was Henry who died first, on 18 June 1872. A friend of the family wrote to Broadmoor to pass on the news, and Catherine was informed. Up in Birkenhead, the landlady of the house where Henry and his two surviving daughters had lodged now took on the remaining children. Other friends took Henry's place as correspondent to the hospital, but no one wrote to Catherine.

She spent the last two and half years of her life in the women's infirmary suffering from a degenerative disease, losing weight and becoming weaker. By early 1876 she had ceased speaking to the medical staff and was unable to get out of bed. There was one last moment of clarity on 16 April 1876, when she rallied briefly on her death bed. She spoke coherently and chatted to fellow patients around her. Then she died from tuberculosis, aged 41.

* * *

By the time of Catherine's death she had ceased to be Broadmoor's only mother. The next child arrived 15 months after her own, on

18 March 1868, and was born to Mary Anne Meller, a stonemason's wife from Newington in South London. At the age of 27, Mary Meller was a short, stout woman with fiercely dark hair. When she became pregnant in the summer of 1867 she was expecting her fifth child with husband William. The Mellers lived a more comfortable life than the Dawsons, in a house large enough to accommodate a lodger and part-time domestic Mary Cattermole. This was useful, for not only was Mrs Meller frequently pregnant, with a succession of miscarriages between successful births, but she was also often either suicidal or homicidal.

Mary's condition was acknowledged but not addressed. Her husband had reasoned that he and Mary Cattermole could control his wife. This was fine when she could be kept in sight, but as Mary Cattermole stooped to light the kitchen fire on 1 November 1867, Mary Meller attacked the lodger, hitting her over the head and then trying to cut her throat as she sat down to recover. Mary Cattermole managed to extricate herself from the younger woman's grasp and ran from the house, while Mary Meller lunged at her lodger's hair and chased her into the street. The commotion attracted enough attention for two men to tackle the assailant and hold on to Mrs Meller until a police constable arrived to arrest her. At her Old Bailey trial the prosecution made no attempt to press her guilt, and after a short hearing the jury found her not guilty by reason of insanity.

On remand in prison, Mary's expectant state was discovered. She also appeared to be rational, so much so that the governor of Horsemonger Lane Gaol wrote on her transfer document to Broadmoor that she was 'quiet and well-educated, betraying no symptoms of insanity'. He suspected that she might be shamming. Nevertheless he noted that she had attempted to poison herself while in his custody.

Despite this, Mary was in far better health during her pregnancy than Catherine Dawson had been. As a consequence, after her son Henry was born Mary was allowed to nurse her child for three weeks, before William Meller came to collect the baby. His wife was noticeably improved since her admission, and though prone occasionally to physical outbursts, was employed regularly in needlework on the convalescent ward. In fact, her change in character had been so remarkable that the Broadmoor staff suspected that it could be attributed to one thing: that she no longer had access to drink. The possibility that alcohol fuelled her depressive and abusive actions had not surfaced at her trial, yet now presented with the evidence, Mary was prepared to concede that it might be so. She confessed to previously intemperate habits, and that she had been excessively drunk the night before the attack on Mrs Cattermole.

Mary's experience was not uncommon to Victorian Broadmoor patients, several of whom had taken drinking to such a level that the courts considered inebriation to have crossed over to insanity. Mary appears to have been one such case. In 1869 a report summarised her as being 'no doubt a bad-tempered woman' but otherwise sane. With a comfortable home and a caring, solvent husband, she was a suitable case for discharge: rational, secure and at a low risk of re-offending. She was discharged conditionally into William's care on 3 May 1870.

Mary appears to have kept on the straight and narrow for a couple of years. But then in February 1873, William Meller wrote to the hospital saying that his wife had recently begun drinking heavily again. He complained that Mary had pawned the family possessions for money to fund her alcohol addiction. He pleaded for help as a man who had lost control of his spouse and detailed his inability to divert Mary from her errant ways. One evening his wife had told the new servant that she was going out to listen to a lecture. Since the venue was one where the couple had purchased seats reserved for each event, Mr Meller set off for the evening with the intention of joining his wife. Of course, when he reached the auditorium, both seats were empty. Distraught, William Meller set off for a nearby chemist's shop to buy some pills to calm his frayed nerves. As he waited for his tablets to be counted out, he chatted to the man behind the counter. The chemist mentioned that he had just seen a drunken woman pass his shop, pursued by a mob of 'a couple of hundred people'. Meller stopped dead: it couldn't be, could it? He raced out of the shop, followed the direction in which the chemist had pointed and shortly caught up with the mob. Sure enough, at the centre of the angry crowd he found his wife. Mr Meller had no idea what she had been accused of doing, and was not particularly keen to investigate. He called a nearby policeman, who managed to disperse the throng, and

William took his wife home in a hansom 'but she would not sit in the seat, and I was compelled to bid her lie in the bottom of the cab'.

William Meller asked Dr Orange, now superintendent, to write to his wife. He said that she took no notice of her husband, but he thought that she would take notice of Orange. As Orange took up his pen to reply, a further letter arrived, this time from Mary Meller herself. In it she asked Orange to visit her. 'I am miserable and unhappy and require your assistance', she wrote. Her side of the story was quite different. She alleged that William had broken her nose, and stated that 'I would rather be under your care than be thus ill used'.

Orange was effectively being asked to arbitrate on a domestic, rather than to solve a recurrence of mental illness. He wrote to the Mellers as a couple. By April the same year, husband and wife had managed to reach some kind of resolution. Mary went on a trip to relatives in Lancashire and Yorkshire and came back more settled. William also stated that Mary had brought little Henry – the child born in Broadmoor – home; whether or not he had been looked after elsewhere until then is unclear.

Although they had another child together after their reconciliation, the Meller family unit did not last long. Mary Meller died on 23 December 1878 at the age of 37, and was buried in Nunhead Cemetery in south-east London. It was another early death for a Broadmoor mother. However, unlike Stephen Dawson, Henry had enjoyed an upbringing together with his parents and his siblings. He would grow up to have his own family.

The Broadmoor staff had now experienced two quite different outcomes for the children born in their care, and would use these precedents to shape their future actions in similar circumstances. Family life was paramount and if possible the children should be reunited with their blood relatives outside; if this was not possible, then it was the duty of the state to come to these children's aid. It was another three years before they had the chance to put these ideas into practice, and this time the mother was Margaret Crimmings, a 26-year-old unmarried servant from London.

Unlike the other Broadmoor mothers mentioned, Margaret Crimmings was a criminal – a convict patient rather than a pleasure woman. She had not been found innocent by reason of insanity, but rational and guilty. She was sentenced to seven years' imprisonment at the Middlesex Sessions for stealing two coats from her brother. That her brother accused her perhaps hints at exasperation with her; that her sentence was so lengthy was due to the long record that accompanied her to court. She had four previous convictions for theft – the first at the age of 18 – and a further conviction for assaulting a police officer. She was a career thief and had already spent more than two years of her life in one prison or another.

The first few months of this latest sentence were spent in 1870 at Westminster and Millbank in London. The prison authorities soon formed the view that Margaret was insane, and asked the Home Office whether she could be transferred to Broadmoor. She was suffering from delusions of a religious nature. Her advanced state of pregnancy was the supposed cause and also an added complication. Before the transfer was sanctioned, the Home Office took the step of writing to Broadmoor to ask whether the asylum would be prepared to take her on.

Orange replied positively, and Margaret was admitted on 10 May 1871. This small, stout woman was now eight months pregnant when she arrived inside the gatehouse. Her skin was pale from her incarceration, and contrasted starkly with her dark brown hair. When she was interviewed, the Broadmoor staff immediately realised that in fact she had merely succeeded in creating the impression of lunacy. Orange wrote that she 'talks nonsense saying that she was frightened at Millbank and that I was the person who frightened her ... it is evidently her desire to be thought insane at present'.

Nevertheless, she was here now and it was rather too late to move her again. Margaret's child was born soon after her arrival, on the morning of 8 June. The first girl to be born in Broadmoor, she was christened Margaret Julia by Broadmoor's visiting Catholic priest. Because Margaret Crimmings was essentially sane, like Mary Meller she was allowed to nurse her baby at first, doing so 'in a sensible and affectionate manner'. But on 12 June something changed, and it appeared that Margaret really was suffering from a case of puerperal insanity. She began to act oddly, suggesting that she had known the attendants for many years, but that now they were using false names; that the nurse helping her was not holding the baby properly but was intending to hurt it; and that people were being unkind and speaking badly of her behind her back. Diagnosed as having entered a manic state, the baby was quickly taken from her.

With no husband or partner to care for the illegitimate child, Broadmoor took the workhouse route and wrote to the St Marylebone Union to confirm the guardians' duty to take the baby. They acknowledged their obligation, but more reluctantly than Chorley in the case of Stephen Dawson, and the London poor law officers asked whether Broadmoor could instead allow the baby to stay with its mother until her removal back to prison. Orange was affronted, as he considered that a stay in Broadmoor would be of no benefit to the infant. He replied that 'the mental condition of Margaret Crimmings is such as to preclude the possibility of leaving the child under her care ... as under any circumstances the child is deprived of its mother's care its removal from the asylum would appear to be desirable on all accounts.'

So it was that the assistant matron of St Marylebone Workhouse came to collect Margaret junior and take her back to central London. The baby girl was placed at the workhouse nursery, Southall School, where she died a little over a month later on 19 August 1871, when she was only ten weeks old. The guardians wrote that her death was due to 'debility', an unspecific Victorian cause that suggested not enough strength to resist the eternal light, though a description of Margaret Crimmings in her Broadmoor notes raises the possibility that both mother and child suffered from congenital syphilis.

Separated from her child, Margaret was pronounced recovered from her mania by the end of August. She became an industrious, diligent worker in the asylum laundry. She was not returned to prison, probably because she was not causing any trouble and also because her discharge was in sight. As a convict prisoner, Margaret's sentence had a defined end date of March 1877, seven years after her original conviction. However, several years of good behaviour and hard work meant that the Home Office was prepared to consider releasing her early. As she approached the last year of her sentence, the Broadmoor staff began to make enquiries as to who might take care of her. Her brother, from whom she had stolen all those years ago, had remained in contact and occasionally visited her, and so he was asked to help. Whatever their previous falling out, he was happy to offer her accommodation at his lodgings back in London. She was discharged on 9 February 1876. Orange paid her fare from Crowthorne and she took the train to Waterloo, reporting her arrival at her brother's house to the Metropolitan Police.

Despite Margaret's good behaviour in Broadmoor, her life outside did not change much. Whatever demons she had sheltered from in Broadmoor caught up with her again and, unable to keep herself away from trouble, she remained a petty criminal. Fifteen years later, at the time of the 1891 census, she could be found spending the night in a cell at Paddington Police Station.

* * *

By now, both female blocks at Broadmoor were open, Orange was in charge, and the asylum routine was well-drilled. When the next expectant patient was admitted it was treated as a more run-of-the-mill event. The case bore some similarities to that of Catherine Dawson, for Margaret Davenport was also a 31-year-old housewife from the north-west, in her case, Warrington, on the southern edge of Lancashire. She had given birth to four previous children before she arrived four months pregnant in Broadmoor on 26 September 1872.

Margaret's two sons had died from natural causes in infancy, but she and her husband Joseph still had the two girls living with them in their terraced house: Margaret, aged six and Elizabeth, nearly two. The couple had been married for ten years, and recently there had been rumours of 'family troubles'. Margaret had apparently been taken ill after the birth of Elizabeth, becoming depressed, and she had twice been found wandering the streets at night. The local police felt that she was the victim of domestic neglect, and that her isolation as a housewife had led to her depression. Joseph Davenport worked long hours as a delivery man, and the family lived a basic existence in the centre of an industrial town, close to Margaret's in-laws but a long way from her own family. The police advised her to return to her native Shropshire for a break, and a cheerier woman returned to Warrington.

There had been no recovery though, and Margaret was still thinking irrationally. After the deaths of her two sons she had become obsessed with the girls' welfare, particularly that of her eldest daughter Margaret, who had been born disabled. One day in June 1872 she quarrelled with young Margaret. The next day, she held both girls' heads under water in a large tub until they drowned. With the children dead, Margaret Davenport attempted to drown herself in the tub, then to hang herself from the banister and finally to cut her wrists with Joseph's razor. Unsuccessful in all these tasks, she washed the children's bodies, laid them out in their nightclothes in her own bed and then came downstairs to make dinner for her husband.

Also like Catherine Dawson, Margaret was found insane without the need for a full trial. At her first committal hearing after the murders she had stated: 'I was very much provoked before I did it. I was made in hell.'

Eight months later, she gave birth to another girl. The asylum staff decided to christen her Elizabeth Margaret. The baby's mother was not allowed to have her child, but she was allowed to see it. Although this was repeated, no improvement came about in Margaret's own condition. On more than one occasion, Margaret expressed the hope that her new daughter would die. The medical staff were in little doubt that given the opportunity, Margaret Davenport would snuff out another young life. It would never be safe to let her have the connection with her newborn that was enjoyed by Mary Meller or Margaret Crimmings.

In line with previous practice, the Broadmoor authorities busied themselves with organising who would take in the child. As Margaret was married and her husband no longer with dependants, Orange wrote to Joseph Davenport in early April. Like Henry Dawson, Joseph retorted that he was too poor to be able to take charge of a child and provide care for it. Orange changed his line of enquiry. He wrote to Warrington Union and asked them to take charge of the child instead. Unfortunately, Orange found an extension of the St Marylebone approach. Gradually, the workhouse guardians' attitudes were getting harsher and harsher. Replying to Broadmoor in May 1873, the Warrington guardians stated that they saw no reason why the able-bodied Joseph Davenport should excuse himself from the care of his only living child, nor why the financial burden of her care should fall upon the parish ratepayers. They dared Orange to provide a legal authority for his request.

As with previous Broadmoor babies, Orange's overriding impulses were for the child's welfare. Though his staff were perfectly capable of providing nursing care, he saw no benefit in having a child begin to grow up in Broadmoor. He gathered together what legal precedent he could find, and wrote again to them suggesting that under statute, the child's legal place of settlement was Warrington; that the father was destitute, or at least claimed to be; and that if the status quo continued then the mother might destroy her child.

The guardians did not dispute the child's need for safety, but they did dispute the extent to which Broadmoor could apply the ancient laws of settlement, and Joseph Davenport's claimed destitution. It was known that he was a working man, employed as a carter, and the guardians stated confidently that a man in his position and his children would be turned away from their own workhouse, should they fall upon it for relief. By extension, they did not see why there was a need for them to provide poor relief to his new child, even if its mother was insane. Indeed, the guardians suggested, if Orange wished to bring morality into it, then how could he deny the risk of harm caused by the removal of such a young child from both its parents.

Orange realised that he could end up stuck between intransigence and bean-counters. The Home Office was compelled to make a decision in the matter. In July, it instructed Broadmoor to send the girl to Joseph Davenport. So Orange wrote to Warrington again. This time Davenport sent a long reply pleading poverty in every sense and reporting that he had developed a bad leg, which meant that he was currently out of work. No sooner had the situation appeared clear than it was muddied again. Orange forwarded Davenport's response to the Warrington guardians, saying that as ordered, he would still send the child to its father, but would be grateful if the union could stand by in case Joseph Davenport refused to take custody of his daughter. The last thing that he wanted was to send an attendant and the baby all the way to Warrington, only to find no room at any inn. He also threatened Joseph Davenport with legal proceedings if he did not agree to the arrangement. This threat finally did the trick. In late October 1873 one of the female attendants took eight-month-old Elizabeth to Warrington and delivered her to her father. She had spent longer in Broadmoor than any of the other Victorian babies.

There were no happy endings to the Davenports' tale. Elizabeth Davenport was another sickly child, and lived for only two years. Joseph Davenport stayed single and never forgot his wife. He wrote regularly to Margaret until he died in June 1889. While her family's story played out in Warrington, Margaret continued mentally unwell; delusional and persecuted. She said that the other patients threw knives at her, and that she was tormented by them at night, with one particular patient able to take on the form of a serpent. She lived in fear and tried to hide as much as possible. Dr Nicolson wrote that 'when spoken to she covers her face with her hand, shuts her eyes and looks downwards and away from the speaker, with an air of intense timidity and shyness'.

By January 1890 Nicolson, then superintendent, was of the view that Margaret could be discharged to an ordinary asylum. For several years she had been withdrawn and uncommunicative but otherwise well-behaved. The official description of her on her paperwork was 'demented' but 'harmless'. It was decided to move her to the Rainhill Asylum in Liverpool, where Catherine Dawson had stayed three decades before. By now, Margaret's husband was dead, but she continued to write to Joseph and to talk to him long after his death. For her, Rainhill was nearer to home, and so on 10 February 1890, she was transferred. At Rainhill, Margaret carried on in much the same manner. She kept herself busy by writing to Joseph and cleaned a little on the wards until her own health failed at the age of 64. For the last seven years of her life, she was effectively immobile. She died on 3 February 1912, choking on her own vomit as she tried to digest her liquid lunch.

* * *

Those first four cases constituted what was in hindsight a relative glut of Broadmoor babies. Afterwards, there were fewer pregnant women amongst the admissions. There was no systematic cause for this or change in the female patient demographic, it was merely an accident of nature. Towards the twentieth century a number of the later Victorian births become bound up by restrictions of patient confidentiality and so there is only one more story to tell. This one came after a gap of nearly six years from the birth of Margaret Davenport's child, and involved the respectable wife of a Welsh farmer, who had notionally both husband and servants to protect her.

Catherine Jones came from the tiny village of Llanllyfni, nestling on a plain between the slopes of Snowdon and the Caernarvonshire coast. It was about as isolated a spot in Wales as it was possible to find. Both Catherine and her husband William had been brought up in the area and spoke only Welsh; neither could speak, read or write a word of English. William was the tenant farmer of Llwydcoedfawr and the generous farmhouse also accommodated their three children and a housekeeper.

Catherine's youngest child, Sarah, was born at the end of 1876, and about a year later Catherine began to develop delusions of poverty. She worried incessantly about whether there was enough food in the house and whether she would be able to afford clothes for her children. The Jones family were comparatively wealthy and certainly wanted for nothing, but even if her cupboards were stocked to bursting, Catherine would still deny that one morsel could be found in her kitchen. Catherine may have been suffering from acute symptoms of a latent illness or a case of 'puerperal mania', as the Victorians described post-natal psychosis. She began to experience hallucinations that her husband was stealing sheep and worse, that he was cutting people down at harvest with his threshing machine. She suffered from insomnia and wild mood swings between violence and profound depression. She stopped looking after herself and would stand, motionless, powerless to direct her own actions.

William Jones took her to see a local doctor, who diagnosed 'extreme depression and melancholia'. He advised a change of scene but no more permanent solution. When, six months later, Catherine lost one of Sarah's shoes this appears to have revived her fears of destitution. Not only was Catherine convinced she was too poor to replace the shoe, she had also heard that a famine was coming later that year and believed that the family was in danger of starving to death.

On 9 May 1878 her husband William left her alone with 18-month-old Sarah for a few minutes in the kitchen. On his return, both mother and daughter had gone. William and the housekeeper frantically ran around the house, anxious that something dreadful had occurred. But the house was empty. As William came downstairs to the kitchen, his wife entered through the back door with Sarah in her arms. The child was dead, her eyes wide open and tongue black. Blood trickled from her nose and ears. Catherine sat down by the fire for a short time, before placing Sarah in her cradle. At first, Catherine said that the little girl had fallen from a chair, but later that day she confessed that she had placed her hand over the toddler's lips and held her nose until she had suffocated. "I would give the whole world to have her back," she said.

A coroner's inquest recorded a verdict of wilful murder and Catherine was committed for trial the next day. By then she had regained her senses and was able to state her own contrition. An array of middle-class neighbours gave evidence on her behalf, leading the judge to conclude that it would be 'affectation' to deny her insanity. The jury did not even bother to retire from the courtroom before pronouncing her not guilty.

Berkshire was a long way from rural North Wales and Catherine was very much a fish out of water. Though some of the medical staff, like Orange, could converse with international patients in French, German or Spanish, no one could converse with a fellow British subject in Welsh. This was a source of concern to the Broadmoor doctors. Orange decided that it was pointless to have Catherine under his mute care and began agitating for her transfer back to a Welsh-speaking asylum as soon as her health was up to it. Orange's problem was compounded by the fact that Catherine arrived suffering from pleurisy. As the summer of 1878 continued Catherine fell dangerously ill and was confined to bed, still unable to communicate her needs. She was not well enough to be moved and besides, the Home Office felt it inappropriate for an agent of infanticide to be housed so soon in less secure accommodation. Orange was asked to find 'some respectable woman, who can speak the Welsh language' to act as a dedicated attendant to Catherine.

As luck would have it, another of the Welsh female patients – Catherine David, a child killer from Swansea, and possibly not what the Home Office had in mind – could speak a little of the language, and so she was drafted in to act as translator. The two women got on well and Orange's problem was solved. The story of Catherine Jones was teased out, her illness better understood, and one other fact obtained: she was expecting.

William Jones, like William Meller, stood by his lunatic wife. He visited in October 1878, arriving with a handwritten note in English prepared by friends. He was found standing at the gatehouse and ushered in. His note introduced him to the Broadmoor staff and asked whether they could point him towards some suitable lodgings for his visit. Of course, they obliged. But William also wanted his wife back and through Catherine David he said so. As far as Orange was concerned, all that stood between the couple being closer together was Catherine's health. By the end of the year, she was beginning to rally, but it was now too close to her due date.

The labour was long, despite it being Catherine's fourth. The new baby, a boy, finally entered the world on the morning of 14 January 1879. Perhaps because of their inability to communicate adequately with Catherine or perhaps because of her previous medical history, the staff at Broadmoor did not feel able to let her nurse her child and removed him shortly after his birth. One of the female attendants, Harriet Hunt, took charge of him, but Catherine was allowed to see her baby regularly while she remained in the asylum infirmary. The child was called William, after his father.

Gradually, Catherine returned to physical as well as mental health. As Orange made the usual arrangements for the child's removal he also reopened the possibility of the mother's return to Wales. William Jones was visiting regularly, and he was also amenable to a transfer of his wife to the Joint Counties Lunatic Asylum at Denbigh, much closer to their home. There really seemed little point in keeping a pleasure woman in Broadmoor, whatever her crime, if she genuinely posed no risk to anyone. Around the same time William took his three-month namesake back to Llanllyfni, the Home Office acquiesced to Catherine's transfer.

It was another three months before she was considered strong enough to make the journey. On 29 July 1879 a female attendant from Denbigh arrived by train to collect Catherine and escort her to Snowdonia. Her stay in Crowthorne, a little over ten months, was extremely short within the context of the Victorian hospital, and an exceptional recognition of the language divide. Catherine Jones's stable family and support from her spouse was undoubtedly to her benefit; perhaps Orange also reasoned that a local asylum would soon see that she was rational and arrange an absolute discharge.

Catherine had received considerable care during her short time in Broadmoor, and this was acknowledged by her family. William Jones wrote in January 1880 to complain about the inferior diet his wife received in Denbigh compared to her Broadmoor rations, despite her notes in North Wales suggesting she was eating well and gaining weight. He received regular, loving letters from Catherine and asked for Orange's help in winning his wife's final move back to the farmhouse where she had destroyed their child less than two years before. And so, in May 1880 Catherine went home. Normal duties were resumed. William worked on the land and Catherine worked in the house as a mother; that day in May 1878 now forgiven, if not forgotten. They raised a family, who were unaware of their mother or grandmother's past or not bothered by it. For so many families of asylum patients this was the situation: they needed each other and were not inclined to dwell on what had gone before.

The Broadmoor mothers represent only five stories out of some 500 women patients from the Victorian period, but they provide an illustration of what life was like across the economic classes for nineteenth century women. Apart from their confinements, these patients blended in amongst the other women on the chronic and convalescent wards. They were ordinary people whose crimes were unremarkable, even if we find them shocking.

This very ordinary quality is reflected in what happened to them after they left Crowthorne. There is no evidence that the medical staff at Broadmoor ever sought to follow up the fates of the mothers or children who had left their care. Indeed, to the modern observer the lack of aftercare is one of the striking features of the Victorian discharge process. Sometimes a patient might be asked to report to the police; sometimes a relative or guardian might be asked to make a quarterly report; with the women who recovered, the presumption appears to have been that once well, there was no reason why they should not remain well, though any new pregnancy should be closely managed. Those transferred to other asylums, such as Margaret Davenport or Catherine Jones, merely became someone else's responsibility.

As it turned out, the Broadmoor babies' fortunes turned entirely on their parents' social status. Nevertheless, they each provide an element of hope. For the babies who lived, by the time they arrived in adulthood they would have had no recollection of the place where they had spent their first few weeks of life. They were unencumbered by its memory and would not recall the walls, the wards or the company of lunatics, and it is unlikely that they even considered themselves to have been born in Crowthorne. The fact that the hospital had no further business with them meant that they were also free to make their own futures away from any taint or stigma. Life always moved on.

8

Escape from Broadmoor

For many patients, the possibility of rejoining life outside the walls of an asylum was a distant one. Though a pleasure sentence did not necessarily mean hospitalisation until death, cases of absolute discharge like Mary Meller or Catherine Jones were very much the exception. Far more patients were discharged from Broadmoor to local asylums than to society at large, and most were in for the long haul of mental health treatment. The hospital could never lose sight of its remit for public protection.

Broadmoor exists to keep everyone safe. We are kept safe from the patients, and the patients are kept safe from us. It is often thought, wrongly, that it is a prison, and equally wrongly, that somehow its patients are responsible for their actions. Yet it has always been a hospital and the law has always understood that these patients should not be condemned in the customary manner. Since the time of James Hadfield, the law-makers have decided that it is better to be humane in such circumstances than vengeful.

Nevertheless, it is impossible to complete a journey around the Victorian asylum without also acknowledging the fear which is such a pervasive aspect of our own thoughts about the place. We fear Broadmoor because although our own thoughts make sense to us we cannot say the same for other people's, then we fear that what we cannot understand must create dangers that we cannot manage. We fear theft, we fear murder, we fear infanticide. We fear motiveless crimes. We fear the thought that we could become sick too. In short, we fear desperately the idea of the lunatics. While mental health remains a great taboo, we continue to want our own irrational fears kept at bay. We ask Broadmoor to protect us.

The result is that there has always been a great social paranoia directed towards the concept of escape from Broadmoor. Indeed, *Escape from Broadmoor* is actually the title of a post-war British film, starring John Le Mesurier as the patient on the run. It is a good subject for any dramatic scenario. Any escape has also been seized upon enthusiastically by the non-lunatic world as an event of crucial importance, and though sadly there has occasionally been truth in that, only a handful of escapes have ever pricked the consciousness of history.

Charged with the task of public protection as well as rehabilitation, Victorian Broadmoor was not somewhere that most patients wished to make their home. Usually, they had been compelled to do so by order of the courts or of the Home Secretary and so those domiciled in the asylum were not necessarily willing guests. Though many of the patients accepted their need for help, many were also sufficiently aware of their situation to object to it and some lunatics embraced this power more actively than others.

Victorian Broadmoor's record on escapes has to be seen in comparison with the county asylum network. When this comparison is made, Broadmoor has a most enviable position. Its escape rate barely registered on the statistical scale, whereas a typical county asylum annual escape rate might be as high as two per cent, even higher if only its criminal lunatics were counted. This was a fact that Broadmoor's superintendents could parade before the Home Office when things did occasionally go wrong. Eventually, Broadmoor's record was exceptional, though this was a hard won reputation after a turbulent first decade.

When Broadmoor opened in May 1863, everyone expected escapes to be attempted. Indeed, the site had been chosen partly with this in mind. Although the asylum was reasonably close to London and the railways, it was also far enough away from other property that it would take an absconding lunatic some time to find civilisation. Escape was also something that Joshua Jebb had considered in his designs for the estate. Onsite, preparations for public protection were made by barring the windows and erecting boundary walls, and each block was given its own self-contained surroundings. The staff lived mostly on the premises, so that they were always to hand in an emergency, and the patients were required to wear a charcoal uniform, marked on the lining with a crown and the asylum's name, which made them highly visible. There were also plenty of in-house security procedures: strict rules about what items patients could have access to; and handover systems for staff, so that no patient should ever be left unsupervised. There were also incentives for the public to place themselves at risk. Shortly after Broadmoor opened, the asylum wrote to the Home Office asking for authorisation to pay reward money to anyone bringing back an escaped patient. Government duly agreed to pay up to five pounds as a reward in such circumstances.

These actions were based on experiences in other custodial institutions and Civil Service procedures. In effect, it was a show of Victorian risk management, though it was not informed by anything as straightforward as an analysis of the risks in this very singular case. Whether every eventuality had been covered would only be tested by real-life attempts, and if the staff had not sought to challenge each component in the machine, then it was not long before the patients began finding flaws in it.

Over time, it would mostly be the men who tried to discharge themselves, yet the very first escapee came from the female side. This came after two near misses from what was effectively still a building site – once from the airing court and once from the wider grounds – before the men arrived. Late at night on Wednesday 8 June 1864, Mary McBride woke up from her dormitory bed in the female block, and went through an unlocked internal door into the ladies' chapel. She then jumped down from one of the chapel windows and ran off across the estate. It had been a remarkably straightforward departure. Not only had the dormitory door been left open, against regulations, but it had been considered desirable to exclude bars across the chapel windows, and once McBride was in the women's airing ground she found only one six foot high wall between her and the outside world.

McBride was a 51-year-old widow, a tall, thin woman with grey hair who had been convicted of theft at the Lancaster Sessions in 1857 and ended up in the county asylum nearby. She was a factory worker and, allegedly, a part-time prostitute. Although notionally a convict patient, her sentence had expired five years before she had been transferred to Broadmoor. After Mary's flight, her absence was not spotted immediately, and so she gained a head start. She managed to make it as far as Reading before her apparel was spotted by a local bobby and she was recovered the next day. Action was promptly taken to prevent a repeat: the attendants in charge of the dormitory were reprimanded, and the absence of bars on the chapel windows was rectified within the month. Broadmoor's Council of Supervision fined the two attendants ten shillings each, and paid two pounds to the superintendent at Reading Police Station as a reward.

This first escape was typical of the opportunistic nature of many, particularly in the early years when human error afforded plenty of scope. So when George Hage became the first male patient to flee, at around seven o'clock on a September evening in 1864, he was also able to take advantage of slack practice. He passed through a gate left open from the Block 5 airing court, sauntered onto the terrace and from there he ambled through the asylum boundary wall, which had been temporarily knocked down while the water tower was being built.

Hage was a young man of 22, with distinctive, auburn hair and hazel eyes, who had been convicted of theft at Leicester in 1861. In jail, he developed the classic paranoid delusion that his food was poisoned and was removed first to Bethlem and then to Broadmoor. He lasted a little longer outside than McBride had done, working in a coal mine near Sheffield for a few weeks, before his distinguishing features led to his recognition. He was re-admitted on 8 November. His escape, though, led to a minor scandal when he confessed that an attendant called John Philport had agreed to turn a blind eye to his bid for freedom. Philport was a prime example of the unreliability of some of the staff during Broadmoor's early years, mostly recruited for their prison or army background rather than competence as attendants. Philport had already been found to be so neglectful of his duties that only a week before Hage's escape, he was given notice to leave at the end of the month. Dr Meyer's mistake was in allowing him to remain on site at all, and Philport carried on misbehaving to such an extent that he was dismissed summarily before his notice period had expired. In between these two disciplinary measures, and unknown to anyone, he had intentionally assisted Hage in regaining his liberty by letting the latter hide under a bed before unlocking the ward door for him. After Hage had implicated the ex-attendant, Meyer turned the case over to the police. They located Philport, arrested him and and in due course Philport was given 12 months hard labour at the Reading Assizes. Hage, fresh from gainful employment, was certified as sane, and sent off to Millbank Prison to serve out the rest of his sentence.

Sabotage by his own troops was a rare experience for Meyer, though quite a few staff fell foul of him. This was a time when the benevolence of the Lord of the Manor came with an acceptance of his moral code, and in Meyer's case that meant an insistence that his staff were punctual, sober and diligent. Staff might be disciplined or dismissed for offences ranging from dishonesty or sleeping on night duty to being a few minutes late for a shift. Drink was also severely frowned upon, and Meyer displayed a zero tolerance policy for staff who appeared at any time to be in a state of intoxication. He ran his asylum like a regiment.

With an establishment that was generally attentive and institutionalised, most escape plans were spur of the moment, seizing a chance to run, even if the idea had been given some thought beforehand. It was much rarer to encounter thoroughly prepared tactics though besides, the level of preparation involved in a sudden bolt did not statistically make a difference to its success. There were also plenty of stifled attempts to escape, with something discovered – clothing, tools and so on – and confiscated before there could be any dramatic conclusion.

As a result, the lone lunatic runner first formulating, and then executing a plan for freedom became the norm in efforts to leave the asylum. It was easier for one person to go it alone than to share their scheme, though the other factor at play was the inability of many patients to strategise. Forward-planning presupposed a rational thought process, where logic could be applied and solutions found. For many of the patients this was impossible. As a result, it was exceptional for patients to conspire together, and only one incident throughout the Victorian period might be described as a 'mass breakout'.

Even then, only four patients were involved: Timothy Grundy; Richard Elcombe; John Thompson; and Thomas Douglas. Twenty-eight-year-old Grundy was the ringleader; 'a powerfully built man' according to Orange; and the first pleasure man to attempt to escape. He had drowned his sweetheart after a quarrel and when he arrived at Broadmoor revealed himself as a man who liked to try and organise direct action, resulting in him often being secluded in his room in Block 1.

One Sunday in December 1864, Grundy and the other men put an elaborate plan into action. While the asylum chaplain was conducting an evening service on the ground floor of the block, this little gang stood in the gallery upstairs, grouped around the central staircase and able to hear events below. They had chosen not to attend prayers. Rather, Thompson, a professed atheist, asked the attendant on duty in the gallery if the latter might fetch a small piece of pie that Thompson had left in the ward. When the attendant went off one of the men waited until he had quitted the gallery, then shut the door behind him and jammed the lock with a stone. With one exit secured, the four men made their way into the adjoining day room, barricaded that door, broke a window, and took out knotted ropes made from handkerchiefs with which they proceeded to shin down the wall. Suddenly, lunatics were raining down the exterior brick and glass. The chaplain, part way through his lines, looked up to see four burly figures passing the ground floor windows. He raised the alarm and called for someone to hurry outside: but an accomplice had stuffed more stones into all the external door locks for the block, marooning the attendants and preventing a chase.

Frantically, the staff began banging the locks to force the stones out. They were lucky. The stones soon fell from some of the locks, and the fleeing patients were caught as they were working out how best to exit the block's airing court. It had been a near miss. A breakout from one of the 'back blocks' was likely to have more serious consequences, and Meyer knew that he had come close to losing four very dangerous men. The event caused the first real rethink of the asylum's original specification. Meyer gave instructions to create an additional, more secure entrance to Block 1 that could be accessed directly from the administrative block. This would ensure that at least one route out of the block would never be cut off in future. The design of the similar Block 6, under construction at the time, was modified accordingly.

More alterations would follow after the successes of serial escapee Richard Walker. A 36-year-old postman, Walker was probably one of the most difficult patients under Meyer's command, though at first glance, he was not an exceptional man: five foot eight inches tall and of normal, if robust, build. He had been sentenced to ten years in prison for stealing two letters. Ending up in Millbank, he was another inmate with food delusions and in consequence arrived at Broadmoor in early 1865.

That year Walker tried his luck at flight a grand total of three times: on 8 April; 21 May; and 3 October. He was unsuccessful on every occasion. On his first sortie, he and another patient, a Scotsman Peter Waldie, managed to slip away from the attendants in Block 3 at 20 minutes to eight in the evening. The only logical explanation at the time was that Walker had somehow managed to obtain a skeleton key, and then bided his time before taking his chance. The pair, still in their asylum clothes, managed to walk as far as Bracknell where they enjoyed a pub meal before being spotted the next day by Broadmoor's gardener, lying on benches at the railway station. Walker was searched but no key was found on him.

He was readmitted, not to the comparatively open surroundings of Block 3, but to Block 1, in theory a more secure part of the hospital. Not that Walker paid any heed to theory. He had developed a taste for freedom, and after lights out on 21 May he began to put a new plan into action, which was detailed in its cunning, yet not wholly thought through. This time it began with pebbles. Stuffing the lock to his door full of small stones gathered from the airing court, he then turned his bedstead on its end and placed it under his window. He stood on it, reached towards the high, small window in his room and broke the glass. Next, he passed his hand outside, whereupon he was able to unscrew the retaining nut and bolt of the centre circle of the window frame and bring these metal fixings inside. Using the bolt as his new tool, he smashed the rest of the glass pane, until before him remained only a window-shaped hole. It was just large enough for him to squeeze through the bars. Walker eased himself through the gap and dropped into a yard adjacent to the block. In front of him was the asylum's six-foot boundary wall. He scaled it, made for the stables and then clambered up onto a horse, riding off in the dark to Yateley.

So far, so good, yet in all this planning Walker had overlooked one small but significant detail. Throughout his escape, he was wearing nothing but his nightshirt. When he arrived in the nearby village, it was half past four in the morning and he was nude from the waist down. He decided to seek some assistance. He came across a local carpenter, William Bunch, who had also risen early in the morning, and told the tradesman that his unfortunate state could be explained by a tale of drinking all night with friends in London. Walker maintained that he had been so inebriated that he had missed his train, lost his trousers (or vice versa) and then been walking all night.

Bunch took Walker round to the village postman, intending to get his new acquaintance a lift to Blackwater Station. The three men sat together in the early morning half-light in the postman's stables, where a jacket and trousers were found to cover Walker's modesty and some bread and cheese supplied for breakfast. However, their companion's appearance had immediately given both Bunch and the postman some cause for alarm, and as they spoke to him they realised that many of his statements appeared to make no sense. They excused themselves briefly to consider the situation. At length, one of them kept Walker talking while separately, a messenger was sent to the nearby Criminal Lunatic Asylum to check that no one was missing. At the gatehouse, the messenger's arrival was seized upon. A party of attendants headed for Yateley, and Walker was back inside Block 1 in time for lunch.

Walker's antics were only ended after one final attempt. This time he had also persuaded Thomas Douglas (one of Timothy Grundy's 1864 escape team), to have another go beside him. After getting into one of the airing courts, the two were found hiding in the asylum coalhole. Meyer was left to ponder once again how Walker could be so troublesome. 'He has long been supposed to have had a key and this alone can account for his being enabled to pass through the doors', wrote the superintendent. He was quite right. Three months later, the key was finally discovered: an intricate piece of ironwork, probably based on an impression made of a Broadmoor key and then worked up for the patient by a criminal associate outside. It was removed from Walker's possession.

This last attempt landed Walker in a form of solitary confinement for most of the next few years. Seclusion was the principal option used by the staff to contain unruly patients; restraint was generally discouraged, and attendants were instructed only ever to attempt it if they outnumbered the patient. 'An excited patient will frequently resist with much violence a single person, but will submit quietly in the presence of two or more', the rule book said. Seclusion meant effectively to be cut off within the block, even if a patient might be allowed to mingle (should he have a desire to do so) at other, communal times. Meyer the disciplinarian was not adverse to restraint or seclusion, and Walker now found himself secluded as a matter of course. Although it restricted his movement, it did not really have the desired affect. His management remained a great challenge, and almost uniquely amongst Meyer's cohort of patients Walker was somewhat abandoned by the staff, temporarily at least. He was an insubordinate extrovert, and at times he practised an attack-on-sight policy. He prowled around in a specially-constructed caged gallery in Block 1, which like some savage rabbit allowed him a room for his bedding and an external run. The other patients were kept away and an attendant was stationed beside the cage at all times. Standing stark naked apart from a strip of cloth around one arm or leg, Walker covered his room in faeces or used them as missiles for the doctors when they visited.

This made Walker into something of a *cause célèbre* for the Commissioners in Lunacy who were required to make an annual inspection of the asylum. It was the commissioners' job to ensure not only compliance with the lunacy statutes, but also with their own guidance about patient management. The view of a man in a hutch did not quite tally with the modern, caring approach to mad doctoring. The commissioners lobbied Meyer to allow Walker greater freedom, believing the patient's situation to be unpalatable and a throwback to an earlier era of chains and punishment in Bedlam. Meyer grumbled and at first resisted. His compromise was to permit Walker to exercise in the airing court, though always alone, and, instead of the company of men, with a collection of pigeons to feed. It was only when Orange succeeded Meyer that Walker was re-integrated into Block 1 society. Orange was pleased to note that his behaviour improved so much that when his sentence expired, Walker was sent on to the Middlesex Asylum.

Walker's legacy to his fellow patients was twofold. Firstly, 'It is obvious that the walls dividing the different airing courts must be raised', wrote Meyer. These walls were not the external boundary, but they did allow a patient to move from one part of the asylum to another without substantial impediment. Meyer was allotted £50 by the Home Office to raise all of these internal divisions by three feet, to around eight feet. Now mechanical help would be required to climb them.

The second event inspired by Walker was the management decision to replace all the cast iron window bars in Block 1 with wrought iron bars and metal shutters. Walker had demonstrated that cast iron was not fit for purpose. It was too brittle and easy to break. So the Home Office took a deep breath and funded that too. However, when the discussion moved on to what action to take with the original windows in the other blocks, Meyer found that the Home Office had reached its limit. The cost of a large-scale programme of window replacement ran into hundreds of pounds. Meyer was told that there was no money available and he would have to wait.

* * *

By the autumn of 1868, it had been three years since Meyer had first raised the question of the windows in the non-refractory blocks. Since then their replacement had persistently been passed over on the grounds of cost. In the back blocks, wrought iron had proved to be an effective deterrent and the windows were now significantly more secure. Wrought iron had been proven to work, yet even so the cash was not forthcoming to upgrade the rest of the estate. Besides, in the accommodation where cast iron was still in place, no patient had used a window to effect an escape in the four years since the male side opened. It is possible that a degree of complacency had kicked in and there were still no plans in place to counter the risk from the defective iron. Now, this lack of action would be seen to be a false economy. Within the space of two months breaking window bars would become an epidemic.

First up, on the evening of 4 November James Bennett, a youth of 18, removed a cast iron cross bar from the window of the ground floor gallery in Block 3 and made his way over the boundary wall. Bennett had come to Broadmoor in March 1867 as a depressed and suicidal young man. He had an unenviable start in life; suffering from mild learning disabilities, and evidently prone to anti-social behaviour, he had spent three years in a reformatory school between the ages of nine and twelve. The sharp shock did not work, and subsequently given seven years for theft in London, he had been sent to Portland Prison, where he was considered to be an imbecile and moved on. In the month before he ran from Broadmoor, he had been fighting intermittently with another patient on the ward and had probably become unhappy.

When he escaped from the asylum, Bennett quickly returned to his old stomping ground in Chelsea, where he had a full three months of freedom before he managed to get himself arrested again, this time while exiting someone else's property with a quantity of linen. Although he gave his name as 'William Watson', he also owned up to the fact that he was wanted back in Crowthorne. The Westminster Police Court officials sent a message to Broadmoor and asked someone to attend court to identify him, which they did, and he was returned on 10 February 1869.

Bennett became the first patient since George Hage to get away for a considerable period of time, and, despite the obvious blame that might have been attached to the window bars, the attendant on duty fell on his own sword. It was considered that Bennett should have been spotted as he made his way across such an open part of the building, and the attendant's vigilance had been found wanting.

Such a neat conclusion was soon thrown into question. Just as Meyer was beginning to fear that Bennett had been lost forever, another two patients disappeared. On 9 November, Thomas Douglas and John Thompson, survivors of the 1864 attempted breakout gang, broke a similar iron cross bar in Block 4. The two men had managed to secrete themselves in a single room after tea, while the attendants were engaged in tidying away the crockery and cutlery. Douglas and Thompson's escape was slightly more complicated than Bennett's in that they were on the first floor, but using their previous experience of escapes they had first ripped up the bedding in the room and then tied the pieces together to form a rope. Throwing it out of the broken window, they both shimmied down into the yard and then up another blanket rope that they had dropped previously from another room nearby. This second rope was adjacent to the airing court wall, so their ascent brought them up to the top of it. Once on the wall, they were down the other side and away. For Douglas in particular, who had spent years waiting since his last attempt, this must have felt like the completion of a long-held dream. For Meyer, it was a nightmare. That evening, he was facing the unprecedented loss of three patients within a week.

The latest two were both old lags. Douglas, an ex-soldier, was doing time for insubordination. Thompson, a swarthy man with auburn hair and deep blue eyes, had been convicted of theft. Douglas was a native of Cumberland and Thompson hailed from Plymouth. Neither having any particular reason to stay locally, they decided to strike out from Berkshire in opposite directions, though it was Thompson who went north and Douglas who went south. The latter walked from Crowthorne to Southampton with the aim of securing a passage to America. He had been a sailor before he joined the army, and wore an anchor tattoo on his left arm as a testament to his earliest career. However, finding no suitable ship in port on the south coast, he decided instead to turn around and head home to the far north. During bitter November days he walked the length of England before, exhausted and starving after nearly three weeks on the road, he gave up and surrendered himself to the police at Lancaster.

He returned to the asylum a reformed man. Biddable and co-operative, he worked in the garden and asked to be returned to prison. His wish was granted in 1870, and he served the remainder of his sentence in Millbank. This was not, though, to be Douglas's last experience of Broadmoor. A little over a decade later he was had up for assaulting a police officer in Portsmouth and given six months hard labour. Orange decided that perhaps Douglas might be better off remaining in Broadmoor, even after his sentence had passed. So Douglas spent the last 20 years of his life back in the asylum's care and died there in 1903 from heart disease.

Meyer's luck had turned, and it continued to hold when Thompson was picked up by the police in Garstang, Lancashire, on 7 January 1869. Within a month, all three of the November deserters had been returned. It was a close shave. It was also obvious now that they had made the wrong choice in leaving all the other windows as they were. Meyer asked the Council of Supervision for permission to carry out the work replacing cast iron bars with wrought iron in all blocks immediately. The council agreed, as did the Home Office, also indicating that they would provide the £1,100 required during December 1868. By then, however, the asylum had suffered its first loss that would not be recovered.

It was Christmas Eve, and patient David McLane was alone in his single room on the first floor of Block 4. No one was watching over him. Before him was his window, complete with its very own cast iron cross bar. To remove the latter, McLane used two pieces of metal salvaged from old locks and a piece of wood to steady the pressure. Correctly applied, the apparatus allowed him to turn the bolt in the window frame. The screw popped out and so did part of the window. Once he was through the gap he made good his exit. Nobody was sure exactly what route he took, but it seems probable that he managed to follow the roof line from Block 4 round the lower level of the administration block, reach the gatehouse, climb over it and then drop down outside. McLane had been put to bed at seven o'clock on the night before Christmas, and was not missed until 25 minutes to eight on the following morning, a lengthy period of time in which to perform his manoeuvres and after which he was, presumably, long gone. As far as the attendants had been concerned, all the lunatics were sleeping peacefully on Christmas morning.

McLane was not the sort of patient to bring about peace to all men or women. A violent offender, he had been convicted of rape at Durham in 1863 and sentenced to eight years in jail. In Millbank he had begun to hear voices in his cell and also to believe that he was under the power of electricity, used upon him by forces unknown. McLane was an early sufferer from electricity, which would gradually seep into the delusional area previously reserved for poison.

It seems that in the days leading up to his escape, McLane had been the fortunate beneficiary of a lapse in good practice. He had obtained clothing and boots without these being checked out to him properly, and then stored them in his room for when the right time came. If the attendants had been more rigorous in their searches, then McLane would have escaped dressed in only his nightshirt, like Richard Walker. A half-naked man in the depths of winter was at a considerable disadvantage, and may well have given himself up quickly if he had been unable to find clothing outside. A fully clothed lunatic had already gained an important lead. The block's senior member of staff was severely reprimanded for his lack of attention.

Delusional or not, McLane had evidently planned his escape well. Apart from the clothes, he had been spotted the previous two mornings removing himself early from breakfast to go and look out of his window, presumably to survey his route. Once he was gone, the same fruitless searching began as had been taking place since early November, but this time Meyer's luck had deserted him. McLane was never found, and his fate remains a mystery. His sentence expired in the summer of 1871, and he was written off the asylum books the following year. It was Meyer's failure, and he moved as quickly as he could to rectify it.

The stable door was bolted when the ironworks on the windows in Blocks 2, 3, 4 and 5 were replaced in early 1869, making them finally as secure as those in the back blocks. This removed one of the principal methods of escape from the asylum entirely, and meant that future attempts to get out from inside a block would have to be considerably more complicated. There remained, though, one final fixture of opportunity within the fabric of the complex – the asylum's boundary wall. Feeling that the airing court walls were high enough, the powers that be had left the boundary much as when it was first completed, which was somewhat short at only fractionally over eight feet. The reasoning was that any patient allowed outside an airing court and close to the boundary was either lower risk, or being invigilated to such an extent that making it over the exterior wall was simply not an option. Any failings in this area were likely to be through human error, and that was another matter entirely.

That hypothesis had been strengthened in 1866, when Patrick Lyndon, a trusted patient, made an unsuccessful attempt at self-discharge. Lyndon was the first pleasure man since Grundy to try and get away, and though he was regularly petitioning the Home Secretary for his discharge he was not thought likely to try any funny business. After 28 years in hospital care, he had lived longer inside asylums than outside them and was considered to be docile. In Lyndon's case, his motivations for Her Majesty's pleasure had contributed to his sentence. A native of Liverpool, Lyndon made the journey south to Buckingham Palace in 1838, where he presented himself as a divine messenger who had been instructed to marry the young Queen Victoria. Declaring that he had "no earthly residence, not even an earthly name", he fought with the sentry on duty at the Palace Lodge and was charged with assault. When arrested, he said that it was not necessary to treat him as a king – and he was taken at his word. He became a Bethlemite for 17 years and was then moved onto Fisherton, where he was considered to be 'an industrious man', albeit one who had also escaped on more than one occasion there. Now, he was in his mid-fifties and worked in the Broadmoor garden. It was in this Eden that Lyndon was tempted.

When sending Lyndon on his way to the garden from the asylum kitchen, attendant Henry Franklin did not bother with the normal handover of his charge to another employee. It was not long before Franklin realised that he had made a misjudgement; rather than saunter down the path to gather vegetables, Lyndon upended a wheelbarrow, stepped onto it and jumped astride the boundary wall. A supple youngster might have vaulted straight over the wall and made for the woods, but for Lyndon climbing over the wall had been exertion enough. He was spotted progressing breathlessly at low speed by another attendant at work in one of the cottages around the wider Broadmoor estate and quickly wrestled to the ground. Franklin was admonished, and Meyer pointed out to him that were similar circumstances to arise in the future, it would be quite clear where the blame would lie.

In much the same way as the iron bars, this breach of security should have served as a warning. Instead it was ignored and so Meyer had his second permanent vacation, when the only woman to be lost forever made her way out a few years later, in July 1869. Alice Kaye was not as fearsome a prospect as David McLane. She was a 30-year-old factory worker from Bolton, with a partner and three children, who had been existing close to the poverty line when she stole a pair of books and two gold rings. She was given seven years inside. Alleged to be feigning insanity, she was removed to Broadmoor in March 1868 on the grounds that she believed she was the queen. As far as the staff were concerned there was no reason to doubt her insanity and besides, she was a peaceful patient, generally working hard in the laundry and on the ward and not presenting many problems. Kaye was as well holed up in Broadmoor as anywhere else.

Her escape was entirely one of chance. At seven o'clock on the evening in question, Alice and roughly 25 other women were in the airing court of the new, additional female block. In the old block, the asylum's brass band was playing one of its regular concerts, the rhythmic pulse of the instruments rising and falling in the summer air. The female attendants in the new block were listening to the sounds coming from over the wall. It was a jolly atmosphere, and some of the staff were dancing with the patients. Sensing an opportunity, Kaye and another patient made their way towards the north boundary wall of the asylum as Mary McBride had done when she became the first female patient to attempt escape. It was even easier for Kaye, as she had assistance. She got a leg up and a push, and from there she was over the wall and away. Meanwhile, the band played on. Kaye was only noticed missing when it was time for everyone to file back in. But then, of course, it was too late, and the vital minutes of song had given her ample opportunity to hide herself in rural east Berkshire.

Her description – brown hair, brown eyes, five foot one and no more detail than that – was circulated to the Metropolitan and the Bolton Police. It seemed probable that Kaye would want to go back to her family. There was also another lead to follow up. Kaye had developed a close friendship with an attendant who had worked briefly in Broadmoor a few months earlier called Isabella Saby. She had, apparently, given Alice Kaye an address in London and asked her to come and see her 'on the outside'. The implication of a relationship of some kind is hinted at in Kaye's Broadmoor notes. So Saby was tracked, visited and interviewed, but it was a blind alley. Neither she, nor Kaye's family confessed to having received contact from the fugitive. The matter was dropped in due course and like McLane, Kaye was written off the asylum's books when her sentence expired.

Though Kaye was not recovered, her escape was the spur to improve the boundary wall. The brick line itself was raised around three feet and the ground also lowered on the patients' side. John Meyer had finally achieved the basic levels of security that would have prevented most of the escape attempts he had endured so far. It was a line in the sand. Though improvements would always be required, never again would there be a lack of basic confidence in the accommodation provided to Her Majesty's lunatics. Unfortunately, Meyer himself was not around long enough to have a chance to re-establish the asylum's reputation for public safety. His sudden death in May 1870 brought to an end his time as Broadmoor's first chief of staff. With William Orange promoted from deputy, there was an immediate shift in tone. Orange considered himself a doctor first and governor second. To that end, Orange had detected a far greater problem with relevance to escapes. He began to take measures against the convict, 'time' patients, who he saw as the main source of all disruptive behaviour in the asylum. Statistically, he was correct: of the 16 patients who had made serious attempts to escape under Meyer's tenure, only four were pleasure men. In this second phase of security development in the Victorian asylum, the spotlight fell on another element – the lunatics themselves.

* * *

Orange had been a member of the Broadmoor staff since the asylum opened. Not only had he experienced the escape attempts of the early years, he had directly witnessed some of them and also knew the history behind the protracted improvements to the window bars and external walls. To a certain extent Orange had inherited a unique institution that had passed through an inevitable period of teething troubles. There was no reason to believe that he would experience any difficult behaviour that he had not come across before.

Nevertheless, only in 1875 would Orange finally feel confident that he had stemmed the trickle of patients seeping out through the bricks and mortar of Broadmoor. Until then, he would also suffer the indignity of reporting successful escapes to his superiors on the asylum's Council of Supervision and in the Home Office. That Orange continued initially to fight against unexpected departures was also down to the building again, but partly down to his more mature regime, with greater responsibilities and privileges placed upon both his patients and his staff.

Escape from Broadmoor

Orange was 37 when he assumed control of Broadmoor. Overnight, the regime at the asylum became more liberal than that of his predecessor. Cricket, tentatively introduced in previous summers, was now enthusiastically encouraged in the summer months. More indoor leisure pursuits were available to patients, as well as a greater variety of evening entertainments. Working parties were introduced to tend the soil of the wider estate and walking around outside the walls became a reward for patients who were well-behaved. In the back blocks, the cages in the galleries for Walker and one or two other patients were removed, as were the port holes allowing the more violent patients to be fed in their cells. Inclusivity was the new watchword.

Some elements of the new outreach were not successful. For a brief few months, everyone was given a turn on the expanses of the terrace, with even the refractory patients allowed to contemplate the green of the Blackwater Valley. When it proved impossible to stop these patients hurting themselves or each other in their new playground, everyone retreated back to the airing courts. Also, while Orange was determined never to use a straitjacket he found it impossible to give up the sanction of seclusion for his more errant charges.

As the asylum was permeated by the smell of fresh paint and the rush of warm air from new heating pipes, Orange turned his mind to the way that his institution was organised. He came to the view that many of his community's ills could be attributed to the lack of segregation between different classes of patient. In particular, Orange argued that the convict class of time-serving patient was far more destructive than those who were detained at Her Majesty's pleasure.

Both elements of the Broadmoor population had been present from the beginning, but Orange now gathered statistical evidence to suggest that the time patients were more prone to escape. Orange also strongly believed that the convicts' disruptive influence ran wider than this narrow problem and that the time-servers were liable either to wreak havoc on their own in myriad ways, or to corrupt the morals of the mostly harmless pleasure patients. His hypothesis was affected by the fact that the numbers of both classes of lunatic had grown since the asylum opened. By the time that Orange took over, the patient population at Broadmoor numbered over 450, which meant that his nursing staff of fewer than 100 were significantly outnumbered by those they were meant to watch. Around a third of these patients at any point were time sentenced, though the ratio of convicts was slightly higher on the male side. Orange concluded that as the numbers continued to grow, so would the potential for convicts to cause trouble.

Though Orange felt that he had identified the building blocks of trouble, the potential escapees continued initially to thwart his thesis. Indeed, the first escapee Orange had to deal with was a pleasure man, and the circumstances related to one of Orange's own reforms. On a frozen winter's day in January 1871, a working party of seven patients and two attendants were labouring to break up the heavy soil in one of the fields on the asylum estate, outside the walls. Isaac Finch, a 31-year-old farm labourer from rural Essex, was a member of the group. Just before lunchtime, having finished his work and by now bitterly cold, Finch asked to be allowed to leave the party to return to his block inside. He was given permission to cross a small bridge, which divided the field from the enclosed part of the estate. As he walked away, rather than make his way back through the gate he seized his opportunity to run, and took off into the woods. Orange blamed the attendant in charge. He felt frustrated that higher security in the compound could always be circumvented by poor working practices.

The man who had just got away had spent most of his life as a member of the agriculturally disenfranchised. His family life had been desperately poor, struggling to stay above the poverty line and support five children. As he had searched for hope and meaning in his struggle, Finch had become captivated by a form of evangelical Christianity preached by a group known as the Peculiar People (the name was meant to be interpreted as 'chosen' rather than odd). Their ministry was an Essex phenomenon, an offshoot from Wesleyan Methodism that promulgated a literal interpretation of the King James Bible, including the rejection of medicine in favour of prayer.

A religiously conservative man, one summer day Finch had been found clutching his Bible 'with the leaves turned down at the death of Solomon and David', the son and father who, amongst other things, incurred divine displeasure through their sexual behaviour. He was covered in blood. Shortly afterwards his wife's body was found at their home with her throat severed, presumably in an attempt to relieve both of them from damnation for their regular carnal sins. He was acquitted of murder as insane and arrived in Broadmoor in September 1870.

Now that Finch had escaped, Orange had a murderer on the run. Orange was fortunate that it was a pleasure man for whom he was searching, as a pleasure man was, almost by definition, unaware of the consequences of his actions and Finch's inability to act rationally was to be his undoing. Walking first to Windsor, then back westwards to Reading, Finch decided eventually to make for his old home in Essex. He tore off some of the Broadmoor labels from his clothing but did not complete the job, either forgetting to remove the rest or not identifying the need to do so. When he reached the capital without food or shelter, an exhausted and hungry Finch asked to be admitted to the Fulham Workhouse, where his remaining asylum markers were noticed by the staff. Five days after he left he was returned to Crowthorne and the superintendent of the workhouse rewarded for his troubles.

Then it happened again. This time the culprit was Thomas Cathie Wheeler, a 48-year-old who had been in and out of asylum care since his twenties. Eventually, one day in April 1852 he knocked his mother over with a flat iron, took up a hatchet and beheaded her. In December 1872, Wheeler was amongst a group of patients from Block 4 who were strolling around the terrace as part of their exercise routine. As it began to rain, the attendants in charge marshalled their troops back inside the block via its airing court. There was a routine for this: the patients massed at the gate and filed one by one past an attendant who counted the marchers back in. On this occasion the attendant's concentration was broken when he noticed that a patient was attempting to smuggle in a stone inside a handkerchief, undoubtedly for use as a weapon. With the attendant focused on searching that patient, Wheeler acted on impulse and concealed himself behind some large shrubs on the terrace. He squatted down amongst the evergreens and waited in the driving rain. Remarkably, he was not omitted from the initial head count when the gate was locked. Instead, he was able to wait until it was dark, whereupon he walked to a point where the boundary wall was lowest, found something to stand on, and climbed over it. Two hours later, Wheeler was eventually missed.

Wheeler's actions showed an unusual amount of consequential thought for a pleasure man. He had escaped in quite a cunning manner and now strode out purposefully to the village of Blackwater, some three miles away. Unfortunately for him, at this point all his fears and paranoia flooded back. He became overwhelmed by the experience. Frightened of losing himself in the pine woods along the route, he began to walk back towards the asylum, intending to find a different path. As he approached Broadmoor he was spotted by the asylum's messenger, who managed to detain Wheeler in conversation until the duty attendants looked out of the gatehouse and realised who he was speaking to.

These cases did not follow Orange's convict rule. In time, though, his analysis would be proved correct. He would be troubled much more by various escape attempts from his prison population than from the pleasure patients. Climbing onto covered walkways, running off over the cricket pitch, or the old habit of trying to break the windows – all these methods were employed by the convicts, and much more frequently than by any pleasure man. It was far more likely to find two convicts on the wall than one pleasure patient in the bush.

Henry Leest's escape attempt was typical. He was a 30-year-old shoemaker from Pimlico who had been found guilty of theft in 1867, but was suffering from tertiary syphilis, which caused him gradually to become insane. In Broadmoor, he attempted suicide and attacked the principal attendant of his block; enduring hours of lonely seclusion due to his destructive nature. Most disruptively of all, in April 1871 he beat Orange's new deputy, Dr William Douglas so badly that the poor man was forced to resign through ill-health four months into his career at Broadmoor.

Leest had already packed a lot into his time at the asylum, when on 14 August 1871 he made off from the kitchen garden in the tradition of Patrick Lyndon. Recently better behaved, he had spent the day digging up potatoes as part of a small group of patients helping with the harvest. Elsewhere in the garden an attendant and a second group of patients were shelling peas into baskets, while another attendant sat on a box nearby and kept a close eye on proceedings. Leest asked if he could go to the toilet and was given permission to do so. He took an empty basket with him and made off towards the closets. The attendant watched him until he entered the building, seemingly thinking nothing of Leest taking the basket, and then turned his gaze back to the remaining workers. When the attendant turned away, Leest used the opportunity to immediately come back out of the closets and to make his way to the edge of the kitchen garden. Placing his basket lengthways against the wall, Leest, a small man, was light enough for it to take his weight. He stood on the end of it and was high enough to grip the top of the bricks of the external wall. He was quickly over it and then away into the woods, leaving only the basket behind him. A pursuit followed within minutes, but came to nothing.

Initially, it looked like Leest might well have made clean away. When he did not turn up, the asylum followed the usual routine of writing to the police and to Leest's next-of-kin. As it turned out, Leest's brother was only too pleased to co-operate with the authorities. This second Mr Leest reported that he had just received a letter from his escaped brother, and that it came with a Winchester postmark. Orange received this intelligence keenly and at once supposed that Leest would make from Winchester for one of the southern ports, hoping to move abroad. Attendants were despatched to Southampton and Portsmouth to hunt down the fugitive. Orange was correct in his assumption, and it was at Southampton docks that Leest was found, six days after his escape, waiting to board a ship to New York. He had managed to find work in the interim and had a week's wages on him.

It seemed quite clear to Orange that if Leest was employable and could operate a clear strategy for living, then he should be considered sane. Leest was sent back to Millbank as soon as the paperwork could be arranged. There is a coda, too, for eventually, Leest was even able to follow his American dream. A letter, probably dating from the 1870s, survives on his file, written to Orange from the distant shores of Cambridge, Massachusetts. Leest reported that he had been shuttling between Rhode Island and Boston on the Atlantic coast. Now he was writing to the asylum to ask for money, because he was broke. No copy survives of the asylum's reply, but if Orange obliged then it would not be the first time that he had made an informal grant to one of his ex-patients. Orange never forgot that the duty of care extended for life.

Events such as Leest's departure only furthered Orange's certainty that the convicts were a risk to his community of generally peaceful lunatics, their influence far outweighing their numbers. In the early 1870s, he began to formulate plans to deal with the turbulent cons. His first response was to take the most drastic action available: increasing the number of patients forced to spend time isolated in seclusion. Many more patients were recorded as being locked up for long hours in the daytime, no longer able to roam. It was not in keeping with Orange's liberal regime, and it was not the solution. His harsh approach incurred the criticism of the Commissioners in Lunacy after their annual inspection, and he recognised that this policy did not suit him.

Orange changed tack. He reasoned that the only way to properly manage the pleasure and the time patients was to separate them entirely. His basic premise was that the pleasure men were innocents who had no wish to cause trouble. None of them had ever been found guilty of a crime, and neither had society accused them of propensity to wickedness. It seemed only fair that they should be kept away from the taint of recognised offenders. But separation did not come cheap, and Orange had to ask for new accommodation to be built, so that he could relieve the blameless. Delivering his annual report for 1872, he questioned 'whether it is just or expedient to permit those other inmates whose lives have not previously exposed them to such evil influences to be contaminated by the degraded habits and conversation of the convict class'. Almost inevitably, Orange was encouraged to pursue his plans, but only on the understanding that there was no actual money available to implement them. He would have to work within his means.

While Orange battled his superiors, he experienced his *annus horribilis* in terms of escapes. It began with the worst experience of all, on Saturday 12 July 1873, with the only murderer in Broadmoor's history to escape and never be recaptured.

On that day, patient William Bisgrove was exercising in the asylum grounds, accompanied by an attendant, Allan Mason. For Bisgrove, this was not a new activity. As a reward for good behaviour he had been allowed outside the walls many times, and he had been exercising regularly in this fashion for the last 18 months. On this particular outing, Bisgrove and Mason strolled around the southern fields of the estate before turning and making their way back towards the asylum farm, pausing only to talk about the chickens running around in a fenced-off enclosure. As they moved on, Bisgrove suddenly pointed out some rabbit burrows adjacent to the footpath, and Mason, a big man, bent down to look in one. Now that he was off guard, Bisgrove hit Mason hard on the back of the head with a stone in a sling. Mason grabbed his scalp in pain and cried out. While the attendant reeled from the blow, Bisgrove attempted to throttle him before Mason eventually succeeded in wrestling himself free. Thwarted, Bisgrove threw off his custodian and made his way, like so many previous runners, into the pine woods of Bracknell Forest.

Mason was temporarily incapacitated, but recovered and quickly made his way to the asylum farm where he raised the alarm, then set off in the direction that Bisgrove had run. A thorough combing was made of the woods that evening, but with no success. Losing hope, the attendants then received word that someone fitting Bisgrove's description – a man with thick black curly hair and a beard, wearing the plain asylum jacket and waistcoat with fustian trousers – had been spotted in the grounds of the nearby Sandhurst Military College. A search party spent the night there. Bisgrove was still not found.

On the Sunday morning, a message reached the asylum that Bisgrove had been seen in Aldershot on Saturday night. So throughout Sunday, a team of constables and attendants visited every lodging house and outbuilding in Aldershot, explaining their business and looking for clues, only to report back empty-handed once again. On Monday, a local woman told the police that she had seen a man jump into the Basingstoke Canal two miles from Aldershot. The canal was dredged, yet nothing was brought up that was connected to the fugitive. Orange contacted the police, also widening the search to include the southern ports. Still nothing. Twelve days later, Orange called off the chase; Bisgrove could be anywhere.

This was another case where the patient was not coming back. It was all very embarrassing for Broadmoor. Bisgrove was quietly forgotten, though his description remained in circulation for a long time. Years later, in 1891, the Metropolitan Police asked Broadmoor whether they thought Bisgrove could be a man called James Sadler, who they had arrested for the murder of a Whitechapel prostitute (and is occasionally mentioned in connection with the Ripper murders), but the authorities were not convinced. It is an inconclusive end to the story, and Bisgrove's disappearance remains without a satisfactory finish.

Orange, a diligent and dedicated man, must have worried at the time that his errant charge was capable of committing another criminal act that would lead to their eventual reunion. For Bisgrove, an epileptic coal miner from Wells, had a violent past. At the age of 19 he had spent his last evening of freedom, a long August one, drinking with another youth and the boy's girlfriend. Staggering towards home, they had reached a cornfield where they stopped. Bisgrove offered the girl two shillings to have sex with him, and she was inclined to accept. They laid down a short distance from a stranger, an older man, George Cornish, who was asleep under the stars, and went about their business. As the other boy sat on a stile beside the byway Bisgrove finished with the girl, got up, walked across the field and picked up a large and heavy stone. He carried it over to Cornish, slumbering sonorously in the summer night, and dropped the stone onto his head. Cornish died where he lay.

Bisgrove and his male friend were arrested and sentenced to death at the Somerset Assizes in December 1868. Both would have hanged, but Bisgrove confessed that he alone had committed the crime, though he maintained that he had no recollection of it. His companion was set free and Bisgrove's own sentence was commuted to life imprisonment. The suggestion was that Bisgrove might have blacked out during a fit. Because the Victorians were very keen on the link between epilepsy and insanity, it was not long before Bisgrove was moved on to Broadmoor. During the last couple of years Bisgrove had become noticeably calmer, which in turn had led to his being allowed the occasional stroll around the grounds. After the escape, Orange reflected ruefully that Bisgrove might have been undeserving of so much trust: 'he was always a morose and sullen man ... inclined to recklessness partly from natural disposition and partly from there being so little apparently to be either hoped for or feared by him in this world'. A Victorian nihilist, Bisgrove's character was such that it seems incredible that he might have kept himself out of trouble for any great length of time after his escape. Perhaps this occasionally suicidal young man did end up at the bottom of the Basingstoke Canal after all.

If Bisgrove's loss was not bad enough, then less than a month after this first unscheduled decrease in the lunatic population, and while Orange was away on a long weekend, the asylum lost another patient. On this occasion it was the turn of John Walker, a 35-year-old stonemason from Birmingham, to breach the staff's defences. He had also been a difficult patient, with a long-term history of trouble. Given an alternative set of circumstances, life might have been very different for Walker. When he was ten years old, he had taken his older brother's breakfast to the factory where the latter worked, seen a mouse, chased it, and then been struck on the head by the fly wheel of some industrial machine. Walker had suffered from learning disabilities ever since and entered into a lifetime of petty crime. The courts had grown impatient with him, so when he was convicted of another burglary in 1866 he was given ten years inside. While in prison, he had begun to sense that he was controlled by witchcraft.

The circumstances of the case were similar to that of Bisgrove, in that Walker was being supervised outside the walls at the time of his escape. On 7 August 1873, he was in a working party of eight patients in an oat field to the north-west of the asylum. The morning had passed without incident, and after lunch the group returned to their labours. By four o'clock, the party had been at work for several hours and they stopped for a break. The patients lined up and the two attendants in charge poured out beakers of oatmeal and water for the men to drink. Walker was one of the first to receive his refreshment. By the time the attendants had reached the end of the line, they looked up to see Walker making his way towards the edge of the field. In itself, this was not unusual behaviour, as the party was some distance from the asylum facilities, and if a man wished to spend a penny then a hedgerow was as good a place as any.

As they watched, Walker reached the edge of the field, where he halted. Expecting to see him undo his trousers, their casual observation turned to alarm as Walker proceeded to vault the hedge and make off into the woods. One of the attendants immediately began to run after Walker but caught his foot in a ploughed rut in the field and fell over. This gave the patient enough time to make good his sylvan flight.

It was a case of *déjà vu*. The usual searches were conducted of the woods and surrounding estates, the local police and their Metropolitan cousins were informed, the railway stations and ports were watched. But Walker could not be found. Orange suggested, perhaps sheepishly at this point, that Walker was a very low risk patient and that 'his liberation at no distant period would probably have taken place'. Nevertheless, it was a further failing. To lose one lunatic might be considered a misfortune, but to mislay two had a whiff of carelessness about it.

Fortuitously, Walker did turn up again, though not until five years had passed, and two years after his prison sentence had expired. It was a chance meeting between two old acquaintances. On 28 September 1878, one of the Broadmoor attendants was visiting Birmingham when he spotted Walker about the city. A pleasant conversation ensued and the attendant suggested that it might be better for Walker to accompany him, in order to officially remove the cloud still hanging over his freedom. Even more fortuitously perhaps, Walker agreed, put up no resistance to returning to Crowthorne and travelled back with the attendant the next day. Perhaps he felt that he had nothing to fear, as he had made a success of his time outside. After his escape, and as the summer of 1873 continued, he had taken seasonal work as a harvester, crossing England on a path from Berkshire to Liverpool. When winter arrived on Merseyside, he had gone back to his old job as a stonemason, moving back to his native Birmingham in 1874. At the time of his voluntary apprehension he was earning two pounds per week and getting on well. It was quite apparent that Walker was sane and was also a productive member of society. It was in no one's interest to stop his contribution. Orange discharged Walker absolutely three weeks later, gave him five shillings for his trouble and also paid his train fare home to Birmingham.

Meanwhile, back in 1873 Orange was beginning to look incompetent. He had lost two patients within a month, both of them arguably through his own belief in rehabilitation and responsibility. The asylum was in a certain amount of disarray. When he returned from leave, Orange was also shocked to hear that there had been a theft from the principal attendant's room in Block 1. Nearly £15 had been stolen by at least one of the more dangerous patients and although searches had been made throughout the asylum, the money had not been recovered. Things were going from bad to worse. The money had not been found because there was a conspiracy in progress. Despite a one pound reward on offer for information, the money was being hidden by Timothy Grundy, a long-term troublemaker, and his new accomplice John Brown. They could offer their own reward, and they did so by bribing a corrupt attendant, William Phillips, into providing them with a skeleton key.

Grundy, who had remained in Broadmoor since his attempted escape in 1864, had found another bruiser to support him. Brown was known as 'a very powerful man'. Stout, 26 years old, and serving a 15-year sentence for wounding, he had already developed a reputation for attacking both staff and patients at Broadmoor. He was another convict who had outgrown the cells at Millbank, and he did not find the regime at Broadmoor to his liking. 'I am weary of life in this cursed Bastille of misery and destruction', he wrote to Orange. He was often secluded in the block and during the summer of 1873 he had embarked on a daily destruction of the fixtures and fittings on his ward.

Then he obtained his key, and his behaviour improved. In consequence, at the beginning of November he had been allowed to move around the block again. A few days later he made out of the scullery on his ward, opened the door to Block 1 with the key and went outside. Then he used the same key to unlock the airing court door, from where he walked onto the terrace, through another door and then into the yard where the wood was stored. He took two sets of steps and placed a trestle over them. Then he climbed up, grabbed the top of the boundary wall and hoisted himself over. He trundled off to Bagshot, where he spent the night in a cattle shed.

Orange could not believe it. He set up the usual detective system, but without much hope of success. However, the next day Brown did something foolish: he used his money to buy a ticket for Waterloo, an obvious destination that was already being watched. He was retaken as he stepped onto the concourse in

London. Under questioning Brown gave a detailed account of his actions and it soon became apparent that Phillips was indirectly responsible for Brown's escape. The attendant was dismissed immediately. A little over five pounds of the stolen money was recovered from within Brown's backside, and the patient was moved onto Millbank again the following year.

Brown's case was closed, but there remained two patients at large. Towards the end of the year an internal enquiry was conducted at the asylum, directed by the Council of Supervision, to rake over the coals of Bisgrove and Walker and report to the Home Office. Orange found little worthy of blame. The attendants might perhaps have been more vigilant, but in neither case were they negligent, and the principle that patients of good behaviour should be allowed to go at large was not one that anyone who understood the subject wished to change. In this last conclusion, Orange stood resolute, reasoning that to give ground on this might well point the finger of blame at himself. Orange also sought to defend his regime further, presenting statistics to show that the rate of escape at Broadmoor since opening was around seven times less than for criminal lunatics housed in county asylums.

Instead, Orange turned challenge into opportunity and focused his recommendations once again on the lack of segregation for time and pleasure patients, suggesting in his inquiry report that it was related to the matter of escape rates. The pleasure man's only chance of discharge rested on his good behaviour, whereas the time man's reward for good behaviour was to end up back in prison – a dubious incentive. Orange suggested that the pleasure patients be allowed to continue as they were within the Broadmoor blocks, and that money should be found to provide a separate, more secure outdoor environment for the convicts.

Orange's argument found some support this time from the Commissioners in Lunacy, who agreed that his two classes of patient should be separated wherever possible. The result was a minor victory, though Orange did not get a single penny of the extra money he wanted for new buildings; rather, alternative accommodation was identified for the convicts at Woking Invalid Prison, Knaphill and adapted for their use.

The next year saw an informal ban on time patients admitted to Broadmoor. Those that remained were allowed to see out their sentences in Berkshire, but gradually their numbers diminished. Segregation was put into practice. Pleased with the improved level of control, Orange trimmed the numbers further the following year. He also began purposely to divide each block within Broadmoor into wards exclusively for either convicts or pleasure patients. It is unclear whether this had any beneficial effects on order, but if nothing else, it does seem to have made it easier for Orange to deploy staff where they were more likely to be needed. Besides which, Orange was happy. By 1876, he declared confidently that the management of the time patients was no longer a problem.

Time patients were sent to Knaphill until 1886, the year of Orange's retirement. Never again would he have to deal with as many admissions from the prison population. It was only when the decision was taken to close Knaphill that Broadmoor became the principal recipient of such patients once again. At this point Orange's successor, David Nicolson, was given the funds Orange had asked for but never received to extend Blocks 2 and 5 and undertake improvements for better security, before the convict lunatics in Woking made their way back to Crowthorne in autumn 1888.

In terms of escapes, the effect of the separation was immediate. Orange was right: pleasure men seldom wished to leave or if they did, generally lacked the capacity to do so. Yet before Orange could entirely relax, one further time patient decided to test his patience, and with a method of such intricate cunning that it completely undermined the sense that escape had become impossible.

A storm was raging around the asylum on the night of 6 December 1874. The wind was swirling between the blocks, buffeting the buildings on the forest ridge. The open gaps between the window frames and wooden doors were howling with each forceful gust. In Block 6, if anyone had looked, they would have seen that patient Thomas Hart was busy worrying away at the wall of his room, inching ever closer to the other side. The catalyst for Hart's labours had been an unexpected discovery; at the point where his bedroom wall abutted the bricks of a chimney flue, there was a much thinner layer of brick between him and the outside world, only nine inches thick instead of the standard 18 inches. Furthermore, after a decade of weathering, the mortar joints had perished in some sections. Lying in his room, Hart could feel the freezing breeze and he resolved to find out where it was coming from.

Hart was a destructive patient, and his bedstead had long ago been removed from his room to prevent him breaking it. Instead, he slept on two mattresses, and this arrangement afforded him the chance to begin to deconstruct the wall at its weakest point. Scraping away at the mortar, he managed to work first one brick loose, and then another. The noise of the gale ensured that no one heard Hart as he was working during the night. By placing his mattresses in front of the growing crevice, Hart could cover up his operations and also place the bricks that he removed between the two pieces of bedding. At the same time he listened out for the attendants, for by now each room had been fitted with an observation hole in the door. He knew that he would be checked on roughly every hour; in between, he could execute his plan.

The patient was a 22-year-old hawker, married with one child; he was also a convicted thief serving seven years inside. At Broadmoor, he had been found to be impossible to employ at any ward or workshop task but had taken instead to feeding the birds in the grounds of the Block 6 airing court and flying a kite for exercise. As a result of these recreational hobbies, Hart had been allowed to keep a bag in his room containing bird food and a ball of twine for his kite wire. These items were about to be put to alternative use.

Hart worked throughout the night at his painstaking task. Then, shortly before six o'clock, he had created an aperture large enough to squeeze through. He gathered up all the pieces of discarded brick and put them into his bag of bird food; dressed in a jacket and trousers that he had previously managed to secrete in his room; knotted his blankets together; and moved his bedding away from the hole. Then he took up the blanket rope, the twine and the bag and manoeuvred himself through and down into the airing court.

If that was not ingenious enough, Hart's next moves were unsurpassed by previous escape attempts. Pawing away at the ground of the airing court, he scooped up earth and sand and added this to the contents of his bag, which by now contained a considerable amount of weight. He took a length of the kite twine and tied one end to the bag, and the other to his plaited blankets. Then he grasped the other end of the blankets, picked up the bag, and swung the latter backwards and forwards until he had gathered enough momentum to throw it over the wall. It landed on the other side, still attached to the kite twine, which produced a cantilever effect using the wall as the fulcrum. Hart secured the heavy bag sufficiently to bear his own weight, and began to climb the boundary wall, gripping the blanket rope and easing himself one step at a time to the top.

He was missed at the hourly check at six, and search parties were immediately dispatched. In the meantime, Hart had begun to walk south towards Blackwater, and he was spotted at half past nine in the morning begging for bread. A local labourer raised three friends, including the asylum's coal man, and the four of them detained Hart on the road from Blackwater to Fleet. In the end he was undone by one small element outside his control. The sole item of clothing that Hart had not been able to hide in his room were his shoes, and once chased, the barefoot patient was soon caught.

In consequence of Hart's escape, the Government's Office of Works was instructed to examine the condition of all the other flues in the asylum and rebuild them where necessary. Also, the boundary and internal walls were finally brought up to such a height that it was virtually impossible to scale them. By the end of 1876, Orange had raised the tops of them all to between 14 and 15 feet from the ground. It was a protracted piece of work, and it meant that the inner compound of Broadmoor was now over-engineered for security. Of course, it had cost time, money, personnel and the permanent loss of three patients to reach this stage, though in Orange's defence perhaps it was difficult to predict in advance just how high might be considered high enough. It could be said that the uncharted nature of the Broadmoor mission meant that all known plans were redundant.

In retrospect, Hart's recapture can be seen as the end of the great escape period in the asylum's history. Of course, it was not the end of escapes – that day never came. The patients continued to make efforts to remove themselves, and always would do, but the successful conclusion of their plans became a rarer thing.

In the remaining period of Orange's leadership, only one further patient managed to escape successfully, and even then he was recaptured the next day. Although David Nicolson rather famously lost James Kelly for nearly 40 years (a story for another time) he was otherwise not greatly troubled by absenteeism. And Richard Brayn never had to deal with a successful escape. Perhaps no one dared try.

As it was, in the 12 years since 1863, a total of 18 patients had been able to help themselves to forbidden liberty, mostly for just a few hours, though with three evading re-admission in perpetuity. This band's escapades directly resulted in alterations being made to the asylum or the way it worked, and the escapees contributed unintentionally to the continuous improvements in the level of public protection. By the end of the Victorian era their absences had also helped to fix the idea of the escaped lunatic in English myth. Meanwhile, constantly evolving and learning, Broadmoor continued to do what it had always done.

9

Only Passing Through

Of course, a lot changes in 150 years. Broadmoor's core function has remained, but the hospital is not the same place now that it was when it first opened its doors. The Victorian asylum is still recognisable, though may not last too much longer. An initial redevelopment project in the early 1980s swept away the extremities of the original buildings, and there are now plans to build a brand new hospital in the shadows of the old. Only the male Blocks 3 and 4 will remain of Jebb's Broadmoor. Such change is inevitable; the hospital is still a working entity and it needs to make sure that patient care and safety are at the heart of everything it does. It is not a museum.

Until now, by far the greater changes had occurred within the realms of psychiatry. Meyer and Orange would be amazed at the phenomenal range of options available to the mad doctors of today. This was not true initially: for many years into the twentieth century the internal workings of the Victorian age were still recognisable and very little changed in the way of routine or treatment. Up until the Second World War, any patient admitted had a lifestyle similar to those recorded in this book. But while Broadmoor maintained the 'moral regime' of fresh air, good diet and occupation, new ideas were being tried elsewhere. These began to be incorporated significantly into the hospital after Stanley Hopwood became Medical Superintendent in 1938. Hopwood was the man who brought treatments such as electro-convulsive therapy and an array of chemicals into Broadmoor, as well as the first talking therapies to be systematically deployed in Crowthorne. It was the beginning of a profound change in mental health care across the western world, and one that has caused much argument since.

Hopwood deserves a mention because he was also a superintendent in the progressive tradition of William Orange. In fact, after Brayn's reign and that of his successor, John Baker, the hospital reverted to the ranks of asylum rather than prison doctors. During his tenure Hopwood insisted for the first time that all his nursing staff should have a nursing qualification, a revolutionary change entirely in keeping with his desire to run a modern mental health hospital rather than a nineteenth-century asylum. For the patients, he provided a formal system of parole, as well as sports and entertainments funds, recycling profits from the new canteen to do so. Orange would have been delighted with such thrift, coupled with the extra opportunities for making industry from leisure.

It was also Hopwood who established the 'Broadhumoorists', the patients' very own light entertainment troop, which kept going for decades afterwards. He allowed the patients to set up their own magazine, *The Broadmoor Chronicle*, invited the Salvation Army onsite to put on regular film shows and constructed a bowling green to add to the cricket pitch and tennis courts. The less athletically-inclined could tend their own patch of allotment instead. The local villagers, who by now had established a thriving community supplying goods and services to the asylum, began to visit more often for shows or events put on by the patients as part of their preparations for re-entry into the non-lunatic world.

At the time, all this inclusivity was seen as an important part of breaking down barriers between the hospital and wider society. It was an attempt to remove some of the stigma from the patient group. Sadly, much of Hopwood's work was undone by John Straffen, who escaped briefly in April 1952 and used his temporary freedom to kill a five year-old girl. This tragic incident had a damaging effect on public perceptions of Broadmoor, and led to a stereotyping of the place and the people within it that persists to this day. Fear and persecution became the default responses to the hospital. Ironically, Straffen's crime had little direct effect on anything else beyond the total devastation that he wrought on one poor family. The hospital responded to negative press by encouraging Ralph Partridge to write a more considered book about its management and history. Straffen's only other legacy is the Broadmoor siren, which is still tested weekly and is regarded by the locals with warm familiarity rather than cold terror.

Far more influential post-war events were happening in governmental reforms to health and justice in England and Wales. When the National Health Service was created the responsibility for overseeing Broadmoor moved from the Home Office to the Ministry of Health, and its journey from asylum to hospital was complete. With the Mental Health Act of 1959 the Victorian legal framework was transformed. A new landscape dealt with 'mental disorders' and 'diminished responsibility' rather than insanity and guilt. There were also no longer lunatics, only patients.

The man at the helm during the ensuing decades was Patrick McGrath, who was something of a colossus amongst superintendents. McGrath went by his preferred title of Physician Superintendent for nearly a quarter of a century, from 1958 to 1981. He took Broadmoor into the psychiatric mainstream, setting up more clinical specialisms, encouraging his staff to contribute to professional debates and inviting outside experts into the hospital itself. He also resisted some of the wilder new notions – lobotomies were not to be practised in Crowthorne, for example – as well as bringing in a more delegated approach to the running of his institution. For the first time in its history, Broadmoor had a proper management structure consisting of senior staff from across different disciplines, all of whom were given a voice and were also expected to share responsibility for hospital protocols and procedures.

McGrath had an enviable level of freedom in which to make changes to his regime. He was responsible neither to a Council of Supervision, nor to the various boards, authorities, services and trust that came later. As the hospital moved into the final decades of the twentieth century it found itself regularly pushed from one quango to another. In many ways, things have now gone full circle, with an appointed group of the great and the good to watch over things, though the modern patient is also represented in a way that the Victorian patient never was. Mental Health Review Tribunals, introduced by the 1959 Act, took away the almost absolute power of the superintendent to judge a patient's case, and the creation of the Mental Health (now Care Quality) Commission in 1983 effectively brought back the Commissioners in Lunacy, but with much greater powers to intervene in patient care.

The result is a very different hospital in terms of the patient cohort. For decades, patient numbers fluctuated between 600 and 850, all still accommodated in the same hierarchical system of blocks that the Victorians established. Every time Broadmoor became too vast, a new version was opened: first Rampton in Nottinghamshire and then Moss Side (now Ashworth) on Merseyside. These are what are popularly known as the three 'special' hospitals. They have always been closely linked, and something that affects one tends to affect the others. All have changed with the new landscape of mental health care. Although they are described as high secure services, they might also now be described as high dependency ones, with the idea that only patients requiring a 'significant period of treatment' will be admitted. This is rather a change from the mixed levels of need that were traditionally encountered in Broadmoor – from the chronic sufferer of delusions to the mother laid low by post-natal depression, who quickly regained her former self.

The typical patient now will have been assessed as suitable for Broadmoor and the aim is less likely to be absolute discharge as progression in due course to a medium secure service. So it is that the average patient stay in Crowthorne is around eight years, and the patient population ends up spread around a much larger number of other hospitals. Broadmoor and the other special services have become a little smaller. Admissions were rationalised and since 2007 all three of the national hospitals have become single-sex: the women have gone to Rampton; Ashworth looks after the men of the north and Broadmoor men of the south. At any one time, there are now likely to be fewer than 300 disordered males on the Broadmoor premises.

* * *

I have visited Broadmoor a few times now. I cannot pretend to know the place, but I do know that it was not what I expected. When I came first to visit, I had prepared myself for something fortified and frightening. I had been infected by the fear that surrounds the name and was quite keen to get in and out in as little time as possible. The sense that I was entering the medical equivalent of a haunted house was reinforced when I walked into the 1980s reception block which forms the modern boundary to the hospital. Security is abundant and invasive, and removed of your possessions you acquire the same vulnerability that an airport terminal provides. However, the architecture of the new reception block is really too friendly and open to cause much fear, and once processed you realise that the building feels more akin to a suburban railway station.

As a visitor, someone from the staff has to escort you. Once you have been screened and approved to go further, you find yourself in an irregularly shaped and anonymous waiting room, decorated with various standard NHS notices fixed upon the wall. It is like an airlock. From there, you are collected and you cross over to the other side of the security divide. You are now in Broadmoor proper. Your host can only take you through each approaching door once its predecessor is safely locked behind you, and you begin to feel the claustrophobic sense of what it must be like to experience this every day, possibly forever. The staff, of course, are quite at ease with the routine.

The entrance walk these days is very different to that experienced by the Victorian patients, and it is difficult to recreate the journey of their own reception. The original gatehouse sits marooned and fenced in within the site, bereft of its former function and now an exit to nowhere. You cannot even get a sense of the generic photographs that are always used to illustrate Broadmoor: that view from outside the gatehouse looking in, generating a sense of mystery beyond the brick archway.

Nevertheless, soon after you are through the modern frontispiece, a sense of the original Victorian asylum does open up before you. There are the male Blocks 1 and 2, for now at least before they too are redeveloped. Block 1, where Richard Walker leapt naked one night and later stalked his caged gallery; Block 2, from which Edward Oxford was discharged, Richard Dadd painted and William Chester Minor worked in his private library and feared the approach of night. These blocks stand three storeys high and surrounded by tarmac pathways and steel fences. The multi-coloured bricks, so much a feature of the buildings of the Thames Valley, still radiate that sense of self-confidence that was part of their creators' creed. To the right of you is Block 3, and through the gated gap between these edifices is the terrace. This still has the capacity to take your breath away. The pathways are wide and the sun beams from the south, casting benevolent rays over mature specimen trees and neatly cropped lawns. It stretches 700 feet wide. The old sports grounds and gardens run like abandoned waterfalls in front of you, while beyond them is the boundary wall, looking like one from a model village. Further still are the fields of the wider estate, where the working parties went to tend the land, together with what used to be attendants' cottages; finally, at the bottom of the slopes there is a part of the ancient Windsor Forest, complete with huddled crowds of tall trees hugging the length of the Blackwater Valley. It is quite a sight; too much to fathom in one go. The terrace sweeps gloriously wide and down and open, like a natural monument to the values of nineteenth century healthcare. Can you imagine such a place being built with such a view today? Our gated communities tend to be pitched at those who have evaded capture, rather than those who found it.

The first time I was invited to Broadmoor it was to scout out the archive, which at the time was stored in the old medical superintendent's office in the Victorian administrative block. We entered the block via the terrace. The corridors now are clean and bright, all creams and apple whites, though a lot of the original woodwork is still present. The superintendent's room itself is largely the same as when Meyer first walked into it. There is wood panelling around the walls, a view over the terrace and an ample fireplace. Here is the room where Meyer, Orange and Nicolson all sat, receiving staff, visitors and patients; composing their draft letters for the clerks to write up. Here is where John Meyer received the warrant discharging Edward Oxford and the one admitting Catherine Dawson. Here is where William Orange received news of Richard Dadd's death and edited the report that spared the life of Christiana Edmunds. Here is where David Nicolson entertained both Sir James Murray and William Chester Minor.

Further along the same corridor is the central hall, which Dadd decorated in such exacting detail. Gothic metal columns sprout from the floor to hold aloft the ceiling, while the stage is backdrop

Only Passing Through

now to a widescreen television. From an adjacent staircase you reach the chapel, to a first floor space as calm and uplifting as you might expect to find in any nineteenth century parish. Multi-coloured brickwork frames the arches of the aisles, raising upwards to a beamed oak ceiling. It was here that John Hughes launched his stone at Meyer, the sound of its crack bouncing round the vaulted space; though it was here also that the asylum babies were blessed beside the stone font. Violence, destruction, redemption: this is where we came in.

My first visit was nine years ago. Back then, I had heard only of Dadd and Minor and had not met any of the other characters in this book. I did not have any insight into Broadmoor's history or its achievements. I was just another voyeur passing through, as so many had done before, completely ignorant of the privilege afforded me of being able to look round England's first criminal lunatic asylum.

What I have tried to do since is to connect with Broadmoor. To immerse myself in the mundane nature of its humanity. To see that mental illness can blight the most ordinary lives. To learn that every Broadmoor patient has a past and cannot be defined solely by one moment within it. To accept Broadmoor for what it is, rather than what I thought it might be.

My own journey around Broadmoor continues. There is so much more to discover and try to interpret. It is an exploration that is never straightforward, nor one to be embarked upon without the most unobstructed of open minds. The more I read, the more I realise how little I know about Broadmoor and its inhabitants. I think that it will always be that way.

10

Sources

A note on the Broadmoor archive at the Berkshire Record Office
Some of the sources listed here are still closed, as they contain records of patients who lived on well into the twentieth century. In these circumstances, the hospital will allow Berkshire Record Office staff to extract information (for a fee) on otherwise 'open' patient case histories. There is a detailed access protocol that the BRO has agreed with the hospital, which can be seen at: *www.berkshirerecordoffice.org.uk/albums/broadmoor*

All references given in this section are from the Berkshire Record Office catalogue of Broadmoor archives.

Books about Broadmoor
The principal history of Broadmoor was published in 1953 by Chatto and Windus. It is by Ralph Partridge, and is entitled *Broadmoor: A History of Criminal Lunacy and its Problems*. There are plenty of details that I think Partridge got wrong, but I am always returning to his book because it is an excellent read.

In 2003, D A Black published a 'sequel' to Partridge, *Broadmoor Interacts*, to cover the period roughly between the 1959 and 1983 Mental Health Acts. It gives a lot of detail about how the hospital operated in this period, though is of less historical interest.

In October 2012, Harvey Gordon's *Broadmoor* was published by Psychology News Press. Harvey's work is a complete history of the hospital, and he covers a number of aspects of the Victorian asylum that I've touched upon, as well as several that I haven't.

Sources

He has also compiled an exhaustive bibliography of Broadmoor literature. My own publishing deadlines have prevented me from making full use of his new research, but if you have enjoyed my book, then please do take a look at Harvey's.

Edward Oxford

Notes about Oxford at Broadmoor were taken from the relevant case book (D/H14/D2/1/1/1), and his case file (D/H14/D2/2/1/96) at the Berkshire Record Office. The correspondence about Oxford's discharge can be found in the Council of Supervision letter book (D/H14/A1/2/4/1). George Haydon's letter to David Nicolson giving the erroneous Oxford story is within a file of newspaper cuttings (D/H14/A5/1/3), and Oxford's personal accounts are within D/H14/D3/3/1/1. Records of Oxford at Bethlem are in the Bethlem Royal Hospital Archives.

You can read the transcript of Oxford's trial on the Old Bailey website at *www.oldbaileyonline.org* (reference number: t18400706-1877). *The Times* also reported the incident on 11 and 12 June 1840 and the court hearings on 22 June and 10 July 1840.

There are various books available on Queen Victoria's would-be assassins, including:

Paul Thomas Murphy, *Shooting Victoria*, (Pegasus Books, 2012); Barrie Charles, *Kill the Queen!*, (Amberley Publishing, 2012).

Jenny Sinclair, a native of Melbourne, has also just published a biography of Oxford, *A Walking Shadow: the remarkable double life of Edward Oxford*, which gives a much fuller account of his life Down Under.

Richard Dadd

Notes about Dadd at Broadmoor were taken from the relevant case books (D/H14/D2/1/1/1 and D2/1/3/1), and his case file (D/H14/D2/2/1/130) at the Berkshire Record Office. Entries for purchases made by Dadd can be found in the patients' account books (D/H14/D3/3/1/1 and D/H14/D3/3/2/1); his closing balance is in D/H14/D3/4/5.

Records of Dadd at Bethlem are in the Bethlem Royal Hospital Archives, and the artwork that he left at Broadmoor is in the Bethlem Museum collection.

Dadd's court hearings were less grand than Oxford's, but there is a brief report of his committal in *The Times* of 30 July 1844.

There are various books available about Dadd. The two which brought him back to public attention are:

Patricia Allderidge, *Richard Dadd*, (Academy, 1974). Allderidge is also the author of *The Late Richard Dadd*, (Tate, 1974).

David Greysmith, *Richard Dadd: the Rock and Castle of Seclusion*, (Macmillan, 1973).

Nick Tromans's book, *Richard Dadd: The Artist and the Asylum*, was published by the Tate in 2011. In addition to lots of Dadd paintings, Tromans's book includes transcripts of Dadd's case notes in France and Bethlem, as well as at Broadmoor.

William Chester Minor

From Broadmoor, information about Minor comes from the relevant case books (D/H14/D2/1/1/3 and D2/1/3/1), and his case file (D/H14/D2/2/1/742) at the Berkshire Record Office. Entries for the many purchases made by Minor can be found in the patients' account book (D/H14/D3/3/1/1).

The Times reported Merritt's murder on 19 February 1872; Minor's trial was reported on 7 April 1872.

The principal work on Minor in print is Simon Winchester's *The Surgeon of Crowthorne*, published by Viking in 1998. The book went on to become a bestseller and is an entertaining romp through Minor's story. It also has an extensive list of sources. Winchester undertook far more research on Minor than I have done, and there are some aspects of his version that I have been unable to verify.

Broadmoor's International Brigade

Not all patients born overseas made the cut for this chapter, and there are also a number of cases that remain closed. Here is a complete list of the cases that I've found, including those that are not yet available:

D/H14/D2/2/1/12: Auguste Widmer
D/H14/D2/2/1/19: John Flinn
D/H14/D2/2/1/20: Miguel Yzquierdo
D/H14/D2/2/1/77: William Stolzer

Sources

D/H14/D2/2/1/258: Joseph Pelezarski
D/H14/D2/2/1/345: Francis Moretti
Johann Kirkhoff (patient number 360, but no case file survives)
D/H14/D2/2/1/472: Joseph Cerini
D/H14/D2/2/1/516: Vincenzo Visoni
D/H14/D2/2/1/541: Jacob Schneur
Felix Mayer (patient number 275 and 713, but no case file survives)
Henry Salzmann (patient number 737, but no case file survives)
D/H14/D2/2/1/864: Pedro Ferrari, or Peter Farrell [case closed]
William Hill (patient number 892, but no case file survives)
D/H14/D2/2/1/914: Joseph Peters
D/H14/D2/2/1/971: Joseph Laraja [case closed]
D/H14/D2/2/1/1008: Daniel Le Grand, or Jean Tallet
D/H14/D2/2/1/1012: David Salewskam
D/H14/D2/2/1/1027: William Thompson
D/H14/D2/2/1/1047: Jacob Metz [case closed]
D/H14/D2/2/1/1147: William Brown
D/H14/D2/2/1/1306: Francesco Poggi
D/H14//D2/2/1/1351: Thomas Cavasino [case closed]
D/H14/D2/2/1/1436: Carl Emil Lillia
D/H14/D2/2/1/1656: Jehanger Framjee Moola Fearoz
D/H14/D2/2/1/1674: Camello Mussey
D/H14/D2/2/1/1714: August Deneys
D/H14/D2/2/1/1823: Francisco Polti [case closed]
D/H14/D2/2/1/1832: Louis Dazzer [case closed]
D/H14/D2/2/2/206: Helena Eimar

Patient case notes can be found in D/H14/D2/1/1/1-7 and D/H14/D2/1/2/1. There are occasional letters from or to the Council of Supervision about foreign nationals (see eg D/H14/A1/2/4/1).

Christiana Edmunds

Edmunds's Broadmoor notes can be found in the first female case book (D/H14/D2/1/2/1) and her case file (D/H14/D2/2/2/204). There are some letters about her maintenance in D/H14/A1/2/5/3, one of the Council of Supervision minute books.

Many newspapers carried updates of Christiana's case in excited detail, and this book has made use of reports from *The Times* and regional newspapers. There are also some accounts of her Old Bailey trial available free from the *New York Times* website.

Broadmoor Babies
The Broadmoor case files for each of the mothers at the Berkshire Record Office are as follows:

D/H14/D2/2/2/113: Catherine Dawson
D/H14/D2/2/2/146: Mary Ann Meller
D/H14/D2/2/2/177: Margaret Crimmings
D/H14/D2/2/2/212: Margaret Davenport
D/H14/D2/2/2/280: Catherine Jones

Their case notes can be found in D/H14/D2/1/2/1.

Correspondence about some of the cases can also be found in the superintendent's letter book D/H14/A2/1/4/1.

You can find Mary Ann Meller's trial on the Old Bailey website. Misspelt Miller, her trial transcript is at *www.oldbaileyonline.org* (reference number: t18671216-105).

You'll also be able to find newspaper reports about Catherine Dawson, Margaret Davenport and Catherine Jones via the pay-per-view British Newspaper Archive website, *www.britishnewspaperarchive.co.uk*. Catherine Dawson and Margaret Davenport's Rainhill notes are at Liverpool Record Office; Catherine Jones's notes from Denbigh can be found in the Caernarfon Record Office.

Escape from Broadmoor
There are lots of places to look for information about these escapes in the Broadmoor archive at the Berkshire Record Office. The following items all contain relevant information:

Council of Supervision minutes (D/H14/A1/2/1/1-2)
The Council Chairman's letter books (D/H14/A1/2/4/1-3)
Letters from Whitehall (D/H14/A1/2/5/1)
Annual reports (D/H14/A2/1/1/1)
Meyer's journal (D/H14/A2/1/3/1)
Superintendent's letter book (D/H14/A2/1/4/1)
Staff defaulters' books (D/H14/B1/3/1/1-3)

This is another chapter where not all the patients' stories have made the cut. Here's a complete list of potential cases:

Sources

D/H14/D2/2/1/40: Richard Elcombe
D/H14/D2/2/1/67: Thomas Cathie Wheeler
D/H14/D2/2/1/179: Peter Waldie
D/H14/D2/2/1/186: Timothy Grundy
D/H14/D2/2/1/232: Patrick Lyndon
D/H14/D2/2/1/260: Richard or Thomas Walker
D/H14/D2/1/1/268: William Watkinson
David McLane (patient number 280, but no case file survives)
D/H14/D2/2/1/294: Peter O'Donnell
D/H14/D2/2/1/388: Cuthbert Rodham Carr
D/H14/D2/2/1/404: John Batts
D/H14/D2/2/1/600: George Turner
D/H14/D2/2/1/614: William Bisgrove
D/H14/D2/2/1/617: James Bennett
D/H14/D2/2/1/638: Henry Leest
D/H14/D2/2/1/640: Patrick Burke
D/H14/D2/2/1/659: Isaac Finch
D/H14/D2/2/1/747: Thomas Hart
D/H14/D2/2/1/791: John Thompson (1871 admission only)
D/H14/D2/2/1/1058: Thomas Douglas (1881 admission only)
D/H14/D2/2/1/1363: William Heaps alias Walter Arthurs
D/H14/D2/2/2/65: Mary McBride
D/H14/D2/2/2/96: Mary Ann Sharples
D/H14/D2/2/2/148: Alice Kaye

Patient case notes can be found in D/H14/D2/1/1-4 and D/H14/D2/1/2/1.

Index

Accommodation at Broadmoor, 13–15, 17–18, 25, 55–56, 59, 76, 84, 110, 129–131, 133–134, 137–141, 143, 145, 157–159, 164–167
Addiction, 12, 52, 86, 90, 115
Admission to Broadmoor, 1–2, 9, 14, 17, 54, 65, 74, 92, 109, 111
The Age, 33–34
Agricultural work, 15–16, 66, 84, 89, 123, 146, 151–154
Albert, Prince, 28
Alcohol, 9, 12–13, 19, 27, 46, 56, 79, 86, 88, 90, 108, 114–116, 132
Aldershot, 151
Amentia, 11
America, 50–53, 55, 59, 61–62, 84–86, 88–89, 139, 149
American Civil War, 51, 54
American Colonization Society, 88
Antiques Roadshow, 49
Argentina, 90
Aristocrats, 8
Armed forces, 4, 7, 21, 27, 51–52, 54, 59, 81–85, 139
Arson, 7, 79
Art, 7, 16–17, 22–23, 30, 37–38, 41–43, 45–46, 55
Ashton-under-Lyne, 111
Ashworth Hospital, 164
Assaults, 22, 28, 77, 83–85, 87, 91, 95, 114, 139, 148, 151, 155

Asylums, local, 3, 7, 10, 20, 26, 54, 68, 72, 74, 84, 109, 111, 122, 125–126, 129–130, 136, 156
Asylums, private, 7, 40, 62, 93–94, 109, 147
Attendants at Broadmoor, 15, 20–21, 56, 59–60, 110, 112, 117, 122, 125, 131–133, 135–136, 142–143, 147–149, 153–155
Audley, Baron, 7
Australia, 32–33, 86, 89, 91

'Back blocks', 13–14, 66–68, 72, 133–134, 136–137, 145, 155, 157–158
Bagshot, 155
Baker, John, 162
Barker, Sydney, 96–97, 99
Barnett, William, 91
Basingstoke, 151, 153
Beard, Charles, 94–99, 101, 104–105, 107
Beard, Emily, 94–95, 97–99, 101, 105
Bedrooms, 15
Belgium, 37
Benn, John Williams, 17
Benn, Tony, 17
Benn, William Rutherford, 17
Bennett, James, 137–138
Bethlem Hospital, 1, 4–6, 12, 30–32, 38–40, 42–44, 49, 65–69, 83, 100, 131, 136, 142

Index

Birkenhead, 112–113
Birmingham, 27, 29, 72, 153–154
Birmingham Borough Asylum, 72
Bisgrove, William, 150–153, 156
Blackwater, 13, 135, 145, 148, 159, 166
Bolton, 142–143
Bow, 73
Bowls, 162
Bracknell, 62, 134
Brayn, Richard, 24–25, 61–62, 160, 162
Brazil, 81, 90
Brighton, 94–99, 102, 105–106
Bristol, 90
British Empire, 20, 32–34, 73, 81
British Museum, 49
'The Broadmoor Blacks', 16
The Broadmoor Chronicle, 162
'Broadhumoorists', 162
Brown, Amanda, 82
Brown, Anna, 82
Brown, Donald, 82
Brown, Elizabeth, 81
Brown, John, 155–156
Brown, William, 81–83
Buckingham Palace, 28, 141
Bunch, William, 135
Burma, 90

Camberwell, 28
Canada, 90
Canterbury, 94
Capital punishment, 2, 13, 67, 101
Cassidy, David McKay, 46
Catholics, 75, 117
Cattermole, Mary, 114–115
Central hall, the, 16, 46, 105, 166
Cemetery, 15
Cerini, Joseph, 74
Ceylon, 50–51
Chapel, the, 22, 76, 167
Charing Cross Hospital, 30
Chartists, 37
Chatham, 36, 40
Chelsea, 138
Chess, 30, 46
Chichester, 94
Children, 66, 82, 89, 108, 111–127, 138, 142

Chorley, 112, 118
Chowne, William Dingle, 30
Christmas, 19, 106, 112, 140
Church, Hayden, 57, 62
Clarke, James Fernandez, 30
Clergy, 15, 20–22, 94, 104, 112, 133
Clermont Asylum, 41
Clothing at Broadmoor, 14–16, 18, 33, 103–104, 130–131, 134, 140, 147, 151, 159
Cobham Park, 40
Coldbath Fields, 91
Commissioners in Lunacy, 14, 43, 136, 150, 156, 164
Commutation of death sentence, 2, 10, 67, 69, 102, 152
Conolly, John, 29–30, 42
Constipation, 31
Convict class (see time patients)
Cornish, George, 152
Council of Supervision, 31, 131, 139, 144, 156, 163
Counterfeiting, 69–70
Cricket, 16, 47, 145, 148, 162
Criminal Lunatics Act 1800, 5
Criminal Lunatic Asylums Act 1860, 6
Crimmings, Margaret, 116–120
Crimmings, Margaret Julia, 117–118
Croquet, 16, 104, 162
Crowthorne, 1, 6, 54, 79, 119, 139, 162

Dadd, Mary, 37
Dadd, Richard, 7, 14, 16, 36–50, 53, 62, 68, 165–167
Dadd, Robert, 36, 40–41, 47
Dainty, Edmund, 54
Dances, 16, 105–106
Davenport, Elizabeth, 119–120
Davenport, Elizabeth Margaret, 120–122
Davenport, Joseph, 119–122
Davenport, Margaret, 119–123, 127
Davenport, Margaret (junior), 119–120
David, Catherine, 124
Dawson, Catherine, 110–114, 119–120, 166
Dawson, Harriet, 111–113
Dawson, Henry, 110–113

175

Dawson, Mary, 111–113
Dawson, Matilda, 111
Dawson, Stephen, 112–113, 116, 118
Delusions, 11–12, 39–41, 43–44, 46–47, 52–54, 58–61, 68, 70–72, 75–78, 83, 86, 88, 90, 101, 117, 122–123, 131, 134, 140, 142, 146, 153
Dementia, 11, 72, 81, 83, 122
Denbigh, 125–126
Deportation, 32–33, 61–62, 71, 76
Diminished responsibility
Discharges from Broadmoor, 3, 32–33, 61–62, 71, 76, 78–80, 115–116, 118–119, 125–126, 132, 136, 149, 154, 156, 163–164
Dodwell, Henry, 22–24
Domestic life, 3, 7, 29, 83, 111, 114, 119
Dormitories, 14–15, 47, 130–131
Douglas, Thomas, 132, 135, 138–139
Douglas, William, 22–23, 148
Dover, 41
Drugs, 2, 19, 53, 58, 78, 90, 111, 115, 161
Drummond, Edward, 12
Durham, 140

Earlswood Asylum, 94
East Indies (see India)
Edmunds, Ann Christiana, 93–94, 100
Edmunds, Arthur, 94
Edmunds, Christiana, 10, 93–109, 166
Edmunds, Louisa, 94
Edmunds, Mary, 94, 103
Edmunds, William, 93–94
Education, 7–8, 21, 27, 36, 50–51, 89, 93–94, 108, 114, 138
Egypt, 38
Elcombe, Richard, 132
Electric shock therapy, 161
Entertainments, 16–17, 105, 145, 162
Epilepsy, 81, 152
Erskine, Thomas, 5
Escape from Broadmoor, 129
Escapes, 25, 111, 129–160

Factory workers, 8, 51, 130, 142, 153
Falmouth, 85
Fearoz, Jehanger, 71–73

Feigning insanity, 10, 71, 103, 114, 117, 142
Finch, Isaac, 146–147
Finland, 85
Fisherton House Asylum, 5–6, 83, 142
Fleet, 159
Flinn, John, 65, 67
Food at Broadmoor, 18–19, 46, 48, 55–56, 58, 84, 126, 153
Forrester, Henry, 22
France, 39, 41, 70, 74
Francis, John, 33–34
Franklin, Henry, 142
Freeman, John, 33–34
Frith, John, 4
Fulham, 147

Garrett, Isaac, 98
Garstang, 139
George III, King, 3, 5
Germany, 37, 68, 70, 79–80, 84, 86
Gladstone, William, 34
Glasgow, 12, 86, 88
Gout, 46
Governess, 8, 94
Government Hospital for the Insane, Washington DC, 52, 62
The Great Chocolate Murders, 106
Greece, 37
Greenwich, 82
Gregory XVI, Pope, 39
Grey, Sir George, 6, 31–32
Grundy, Timothy, 132–133, 135, 155
Gull, William, 102–103
Guyana, 81

HMPs (see pleasure patients)
HMS Pinafore, 16
HMS Suffolk, 33
Hackney, 74
Hadfield, James, 3–5, 8, 9, 12, 128
Hage, George, 131–132, 138
Hanging see capital punishment
Hanwell Asylum, 29, 74
Hardy, Gathorne, 32
Hart, Thomas, 157–159
Haydon, George, 32–33, 43–45
Hayter, William, 31–32

Index

Heelas' Department Store, 33
Heidelberg University, 20
Heim, Peter, 68
Hennessy, Steve, 106
Hill, William, 85
Hodgkin, Thomas, 29–30
Holborn, 53
Home Office, 6, 20, 41, 71, 78, 85, 102, 105, 109, 117, 121, 124–125, 129–130, 137, 140, 144, 156, 163
Home Secretary, 3, 10, 31–32, 102, 129
Hong Kong, 86
Hopwood, Stanley, 161–162
Hood, Charles, 31, 43–44
Horsemonger Lane Gaol, 114
Houlton, George, 7
Hounslow, 27
Hughes, John, 22, 167
Hunt, Harriet, 125
Hunter, Archibald, 72
Hysteria, 94, 103

Illegitimacy, 2, 86, 89, 118
Imbeciles (see learning disability)
India, 68, 71–72, 89–90
Infanticide, 8, 111, 120, 124, 128
Iran, 73
Ireland, 76, 110
Isaac, John Baldwin, 24, 67
Italy, 37, 39, 74–78, 85

Jebb, Joshua, 6, 129, 161
Joint Counties Asylum, 125–126
Jones, Catherine, 123–128
Jones, Sarah, 123–124
Jones, William, 123–126
Jones, William (junior), 125–126

Kaye, Alice, 142–143
Kelly, James, 160
Kingston-upon-Thames, 54
Kirchoff, Wilhelm, 84–85
Kirkdale Prison, 68
Knaphill Prison, 156–157
Knight, Adelaide, 82

Lambeth, 27
Lancaster, 139

The Lancet, 30
Languages, 30, 65, 67, 69, 71, 73–74, 77, 84, 123–125
Le Mesurier, John, 129
Learning disabilities, 2, 11, 94, 137–138, 153
Leest, Henry, 148–150
Leicester, 131
Lewes, 99, 101, 103–104
Liberia, 88–89
Lights and Shadows of Melbourne Life, 34
Lillia, Carl, 85
Liverpool, 68, 89–90, 111–112, 122, 141, 154
Llanllyfni, 123, 125
London, 1, 3, 12, 22, 27, 38, 40, 45, 53–54, 57, 64–65, 68–69, 71–77, 82–84, 89–91, 97, 99–101, 113, 116–117, 119, 138, 141, 143, 147, 156
London County Council, 17
Lyndon, Patrick, 141–142, 148
Lyons, James, 22

McBride, Mary, 130–131, 143
McGrath, Patrick, 56, 163
McLane, David, 140–141
Maclean, Roderick, 34
McNaughten Rules, 12, 100
McNaughten, Daniel, 12
Madame Tussaud's, 29
Maida Vale, 72
Malta, 38
Manchester, 111
Mania, 11, 29, 42, 66–69, 73, 77, 85, 111–113, 118, 123
Margate, 93, 97
Marriage, 27, 51, 75, 79, 81, 86, 95, 109–110, 115–116, 119, 123, 126, 146, 158
Marshall Hall, Edward, 106
Martin, Lord, 101
Marylebone, 118, 120
Mason, Allan, 150–151
Massey, Anna, 106
Master of the Rolls, 22
Masturbation, 9, 51
Maudsley, Henry, 100

May, Adam, 98
Mayer, Felix, 79–80
Mayer, Matthew, 79
Maynard, J.G., 96, 98–100
Media reaction to Broadmoor patients, 12, 29, 92–93, 99–100, 162
Medicines (see Drugs)
Melancholia, 11, 39, 42, 75, 80–81, 119–120, 123
Melbourne, 32–34
Meller, Henry, 114–116
Meller, Mary Ann, 113–117, 120, 128
Meller, William, 114–116, 125
Menopause, 108
Mental deficiency (see learning disabilities)
Mental Health Act 1959, 163
Mental Health Commission, 164
Merritt, Eliza, 60–61
Merritt, George, 53–54, 60
Mersey, river, 68, 112
Meyer, John, 20–23, 31, 76, 84, 112, 131–133, 135–139, 142–144, 161, 166
Midland Perambulator Company, 72
Military courts, 7
Millbank Prison, 69, 71, 117, 132, 134, 139–140, 149, 155–156
Miller, Charles, 96
Millwall Docks, 76
Ministry of Health, 163
Minor, Alfred, 61–62
Minor, Eastman, 50–51
Minor, George, 52–53
Minor, Lucy, 50
Minor, William Chester, 14, 16, 50–63, 69, 83, 165–167
Monomania, 11, 44, 52, 58
Moral insanity, 11, 96, 99–100, 102, 104–105, 152–153
Moral treatment, 2–3, 15–16, 30, 78, 80, 110, 161
Moretti, Elizabeth, 75
Moretti, Francisco, 74–78
Moss Side Hospital, 164
Murder, 2, 8, 13, 40, 53, 66, 68, 73, 75, 81, 96, 108, 111, 120, 124, 128, 132, 146–147, 152, 162

Murray, James, 56–58, 60, 62–63, 166
Music, 16, 30, 55–56, 143

National Health Service, 163
Newbury, 79
Newgate Prison, 5, 29, 88, 99, 101
Newington, 113
Nicholson, Margaret, 4
Nicolson, David, 16, 22, 24–25, 33, 47, 56–59, 105, 122, 157, 160, 166
Nottingham, 2

Occupational therapy, 2, 15, 30–31, 42–43, 45, 55–57, 69, 75, 79–80, 105, 110, 114, 118, 122, 142, 145–146, 153, 158, 161
Office of Works, 159
Ogilvy, Alexander, 86–89
Old Bailey, 29, 72, 77, 88, 99–101, 114
Orange, William, 20, 22–25, 46, 55, 59–60, 71, 73, 79, 88, 91, 102–105, 116–121. 124–126, 136, 139, 144–157, 159–162, 166
Orr, William, 87–88
Osiris, 39, 47
Oxford, 57
Oxford English Dictionary, 50, 56–57
Oxford University Press, 63
Oxford, Edward, 7–8, 14, 26–35, 37, 42, 165–166
Oxford, Hannah, 27, 29

Paddington, 119
Palestine, 38
Paranoia, 38, 44, 53–54, 75, 79, 84, 86–87, 90–91, 112, 122, 131, 148
Parkhurst Prison, 72
Parr, Mary Ann, 2, 10
Parsee, 73
Partridge, Ralph, 162
Payments to patients, 23, 46, 55, 59
Peckham, 94
Peculiar People, 146
Peel, Robert, 12
Pelezarski, Joseph, 83–84
Personality disorder (see Moral insanity)

178

Index

Peters, Joseph, 88–92
Phelps, Charles, 16, 33
Phelps, Florence, 16
Phillips, Thomas, 37–39
Phillips, William, 155
Philport, John, 131–132
Pimlico, 148
Pleasure patients, 8–9, 13, 30, 45, 54, 65, 67, 73–92, 102, 108–109, 111, 114, 125, 141, 144–148, 156
Plymouth, 33, 139
Poaching, 2, 66
Poggi, Francesco, 85
Poisons, 58, 86, 93, 95–98, 100, 114, 131
Poland, 73, 83
Police, 29, 32, 53, 70, 77, 90, 96–98, 114–115, 111, 119, 126, 131, 139, 143, 151, 154
Portland Prison, 138
Portsmouth, 24, 139, 149
Poverty, 2, 9, 112, 121, 142, 146
Pregnancy and childbirth, 9, 12, 101, 105, 108–127
Prisons, 3, 5, 10, 21, 24, 29, 68–69, 71–72, 88, 90–91, 99, 101, 109, 114, 117–118, 132, 139–140, 149, 153, 155–157
Prostitution, 7, 52, 130
Psychiatry, 2, 29–30, 36, 108, 161–163
Psychopaths (see moral insanity)
Puberty, 108
Puerperal psychosis, 105, 117, 123
Purgatives, 78

Racism, 76, 92
Railways, 1, 6, 17, 34, 62, 79, 97–98, 119, 134, 154–155
Rainhill Asylum, 68, 111, 122
Rampton Hospital, 164
Reading, 33, 79, 84, 91, 131, 147
Refractory blocks (see back blocks)
Religion, 4, 9, 12, 15, 19–22, 39, 41, 44–45, 47, 50, 73, 75, 133, 142, 146
Restraint, 21, 42, 135, 145
Retreat for the Elderly Insane, Connecticut, 62
Ripper murders, 152
Rochester, 36–37

Royal Academy, 37
Rudall Carte, 55
Russia, 69–71, 73–74, 83, 85

SS Durham, 91
SS Peru, 86–87
St Albans, 66
St Luke's Hospital, London, 40
St Pancras Station, 62
Saby, Isabella, 143
Sadler, James, 152
Sailors and sailing, 67–68, 81–82, 85–92, 139
Salewskam, David, 73–74
Salisbury, 5, 83
Salvation Army, 162
Sandhurst Military College, 151
Schizophrenia, 54
Schneur, Jacob, 69–72, 78
Scotland, 96
Seclusion, 22, 24, 66, 133, 135–136, 150, 155
Sedatives, 2, 78
Servants, 8, 56, 97, 109, 115–116, 123
Sex, sex crimes and sexuality, 8, 51–53, 55, 60–61, 90, 94–95, 98, 104–105, 107, 140, 152
Sheerness, 81
Sheffield, 131
Sheppey, 82
Shoemakers, 15, 68–69, 79–80, 148
Sierra Leone, 89
Singapore, 51
Sittingbourne, 81
Southall, 93, 118
Southampton, 139, 149
Southport, 105
Southwark, 1, 30, 65
Spain, 66
Staff at Broadmoor, 16–17, 19–25, 48, 56, 58, 103, 110, 129–130, 133, 135, 141, 146, 148, 155, 161–163, 166
Stolzer, William, 65, 68–69
Straffen, John, 162–163
Suicide, 8, 84–85, 137, 148
The Surgeon of Crowthorne, 50
Surgery, 51, 55, 75, 81, 90–92
Sutherland, Alexander, 40

179

Swansea, 124
Switzerland, 37, 65
Syphilis, 2, 72, 118, 148
Syria, 38

Tailors, 15, 73, 75
Tamils, 50
Tartary, 70
Tasmania, 20, 34
Tate Britain, 48
Tennis, 162
Terrace, the, 13–14, 104, 110, 131, 145, 147, 155, 166
Terrorism, 28–29, 66, 77
Thames, river, 2, 76
Theatre Royal, Drury Lane, 3–4
Theft, 1, 8, 65–66, 68, 72, 85, 89, 108, 117, 128, 130–131, 134, 138–139, 142, 148, 153, 155, 158
Thompson, John, 132–133, 138–139
Thompson, William, 85–88
Tilbury Docks, 62
Time patients, 10, 65–72, 108, 116, 118, 130–131, 133, 139–140, 143–146, 148–158
The Times, 99–100, 102
Tobacco, 19, 55, 67, 74
Tourism, 37–39, 53, 96
Transportation, 2, 32, 33, 69
Treason, 4, 8, 26, 28, 33
Trinidad, 90
Tuberculosis, 48, 50, 55, 113
Tuchet, William Ross, 7–9
Turkey, 37, 83

Unfit to plead (insane on arraignment), 42, 68, 73, 77, 111, 120

Vagrancy, 8, 66
Victor Emmanuel, King of Italy, 77
Victoria, Princess Royal, 28

Victoria, Queen, 8, 19, 25–26, 28, 31, 34, 84, 142
Victoria Station, 97–98
Visits, 17, 58–59, 62, 69, 76, 79, 82, 113–114, 125
Visoni, Vicenzo, 76–78

Waldie, Peter, 134
Wales, 37, 123–126
Walker, John, 153–154, 156
Walker, Richard, 133–137, 140, 145
Wandsworth, 20
Warrington, 119–122
Wars, Crimean, 20, 83
Wars, French Revolutionary, 3
Waterloo Station, 1, 53, 62, 119, 155
Wellington College, 6
Wells, 152
Westminster, 65, 117, 138
Wheeler, Richard, 45
Wheeler, Thomas Cathie, 147–148
Wicked Women, 106
Widmer, Auguste, 65–66
Wigwam Shipowners, 91
Winchester, 149
Winchester, Simon, 50, 57, 60–61, 63
Windsor, 34, 147
Windsor Forest, 1, 6, 166
Woking, 156–157
Wokingham, 1, 65
Wood, William, 100
Woolwich Arsenal, 82
Workhouses, 73, 77, 82, 109, 111–113, 118, 120–121, 147
Wormwood Scrubs Prison, 72

Yale University, 51
Yateley, 134–135
York, 2
'Young England', 27
Yzquierdo, Miguel, 65–67, 77

Delve deeper into the world of the nineteenth century asylum in Mark Stevens' next book

The Victorian Asylum: A Patient's Handbook

Would you like to take another tour of the Victorian asylum?

Mark Stevens reveals what everyday life was really like for the thousands of men, women and children admitted to lunatic asylums all over Britain during the 1800s. Unlocking the secrets held in asylum archives, Mark recreates the experiences of a new patient leaving society and entering asylum care, perhaps for a lifetime.

Discover from a patient's perspective what it was really like to stay in one of these infamous institutions. How were people admitted – and how did they get out? Who were the staff? What sort of treatments did patients receive? What was their legal position? Were Victorian asylums really the grim places that we might imagine them to be?

In a special research section Mark also shares his expertise as a professional archivist. Do you have an ancestor who was admitted to a Victorian asylum? If so, discover how to unlock the truth about the life of a lunatic in nineteenth century Britain.

Published by Pen and Sword Books in autumn 2014.